Functional Outcomes

Documentation for Rehabilitation

Functional Outcomes

Documentation for Rehabilitation

Lori Quinn, EdD, PT
Associate Professor
Program in Physical Therapy
New York Medical College
Valhalla, New York

James Gordon, EdD, PT
Associate Professor and Chair
Department of Biokinesiology and Physical Therapy
University of Southern California
Los Angeles, California

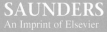
SAUNDERS
An Imprint of Elsevier

SAUNDERS
An Imprint of Elsevier

11830 Westline Industrial Drive
St. Louis, Missouri 63146

NOTICE

Physical Therapy is an ever-changing field. Standard safety precautions must be followed, but as new research and clinical experience broaden our knowledge, changes in treatment and drug therapy may become necessary or appropriate. Readers are advised to check the most current product information provided by the manufacturer of each drug to be administered to verify the recommended dose, the method and duration of administration, and contraindications. It is the responsibility of the licensed prescriber relying on experience and knowledge of the patient, to determine dosages and the best treatment for each individual patient. Neither the publisher nor the author assume any liability for any injury and/or damage to persons or property arising from this publication.

The Publisher

International Standard Book Number 0-7216-8947-7

Acquisitions Editor: Marion Waldman
Developmental Editor: Marjory Fraser
Publishing Services Manager: Pat Joiner
Senior Designer: Mark A. Oberkrom
Interior Design: Judith A. Schmitt

Printed in the United States of America.

Last digit is the print number: 9   8   7   6   5   4   3   2

Contributors

JODY FELD, MS, PT
Clinical Faculty Associate
New York Medical College;
Supervisor of Inpatient Spinal Cord Injury
    and Brain Injury
Burke Rehabilitation Center
White Plains, New York

JANET HERBOLD, MA, PT
Director of Rehabilitation Services
Burke Rehabilitation Hospital
White Plains, New York

KAREN D. STUTMAN, MS, PT, ATC
Clinical Faculty Associate
New York Medical College;
Part-Time Staff Therapist
Wilton Physical Therapy
Wilton, Connecticut

Reviewers

NANCEY A. BOOKSTEIN, EdD, PT
University of Colorado Health Sciences Center
Denver, Colorado

PATRICIA R. CURRATTI, PT, MS, PCS
Assistant Clinical Professor
University of Michigan—Flint
Flint, Michigan

APRIL FRIEDMAN, PT, MS
Assistant Professor
The Sage College
Troy, New York

REBECCA GRAVES, MS, PT
Program Coordinator
Whatcom Community College
Bellingham, Washington

SUSAN HOWARD, PT
PTA Program Director
Riverland Community College
Albert Lea, Minnesota

DAVID A. LAKE, PT, PhD
Professor and Department Head
Armstrong Atlantic State University
Savannah, Georgia

SUSAN M. ROEHRIG, PT, PhD
Professor
Hardin-Simmons University
Abilene, Texax

To Gram, my first teacher of documentation, for your loving spirit
L.Q.

To Dr. Robert Gordon, my father, whose dedication to the art and science of patient care has always been my primary source of inspiration
J.G.

Preface

This book was born out of necessity. It began its life, in a rudimentary form, as a teaching manual for students in the physical therapy program at New York Medical College. We needed a textbook that would provide a framework for functional outcomes documentation, and no satisfactory texts existed. So we wrote one.

The main philosophical idea underlying this textbook is simple: not only is the logic of clinical reasoning reflected in documentation, but documentation itself shapes the process of clinical reasoning. Thus, we would argue, one of the best ways to teach clinical reasoning skills is by teaching a careful and systematic approach to documentation. This book is therefore not just a "how-to" book on documentation of physical therapy practice. Rather, it presents a framework for clinical reasoning based on a disablement model, specifically the Nagi model.

The terms *disability, functional limitations, impairments,* and *pathology* are now incorporated into the vocabularies of contemporary physical therapists and certainly of entry-level physical therapy students. Nevertheless, for physical therapists to "walk the walk" rather than just "talk the talk," the disablement framework exemplified by the Nagi model must be incorporated into how they design and implement evaluations and interventions. This process is reflected in the documentation written by physical therapists. The outside world views physical therapy primarily by words that are written—as communicated in a medical record, progress notes given to a patient or doctor, or forms completed for an insurance company. We believe that documentation shapes *and* reflects the advances in the science of physical therapy and therefore requires an updated framework that incorporates current knowledge regarding the disablement and rehabilitation processes.

The purpose of this book is to provide a general approach to documentation—not a rigid format. It is, first and foremost, a textbook for entry-level physical therapist and physical therapist assistant students. It is intended to promote a style and philosophy of documentation that can be used throughout an entire physical therapy curriculum. However, it is also a book that

we hope will appeal to practicing physical therapists and physical therapist assistants who are searching for a better structure for the note-writing process. We have provided examples and exercises related to wide-ranging areas of physical therapy practice, including pediatrics, rehabilitation, women's health, health and wellness, orthopedics, and acute care. This book was designed to assist students and therapists to organize their clinical reasoning and establish a framework for documentation that is easily adaptable to different practice settings and patient populations. Although this book has many examples and exercises, it certainly does not include all possible types of documentation or all details of how you would document in different settings. Rather, this book provides a method for learning good documentation skills that can be adapted to different settings.

Although physical therapist assistants and physical therapist assistant students will find this book relevant, their practice is inherently limited to writing of daily or per session notes. A large portion of this book focuses on documentation of the initial evaluation. However, the components listed in each of these chapters, particularly documentation of functional skills, are important components of the daily note documentation.

The book is divided into three sections. The first section provides the overall theoretical framework. The second section explains in detail each of the specific components of a functional outcomes initial evaluation and provides extensive examples and practice. The third section considers other types of documentation, such as progress notes and letters to third parties.

We believe that a standardized format for documentation should be introduced early in a physical therapy curriculum so that students can practice writing notes in successive clinical courses. Furthermore, we have structured the book so that students should be able to learn the approach on their own without requiring a separate course on documentation. Thus we have provided many opportunities for practice of documentation skills through exercises at the end of most chapters. Nevertheless, the book will work best when an instructor is guiding the learning process and available to answer questions. The exercises are written primarily for physical therapist students and physical therapist assistant students in entry-level education. However, depending on their level of education and the design of the curriculum, many students may not be able to complete all of the exercises. This is particularly true for those exercises in which the reader is asked to rewrite problematic documentation. Some students may only have limited knowledge to be able to rewrite the statements accurately.

As much as possible, we have attempted to incorporate the terminology and main ideas of the *Guide to Physical Therapist Practice*. For the most part, they are very relevant to and consistent with functional outcomes and documentation. Readers should find this book *"Guide*-friendly," and we have reprinted figures and adapted components of the *Guide* into our documentation framework.

Readers will note that although the *Guide* uses the term "patient/client" to denote those individuals served by PTs, we have chosen to use only the term "patient." This is solely for ease and consistency, although we recognize the importance of the differentiation of these two terms in PT vocabulary.

This book should be used in conjunction with other resources and references related to functional outcomes and documentation. Many of these resources are listed in the back of this book. In particular, there are important legal aspects of documentation. We have provided a foundation for key elements related to legal aspects of documentation; however, readers should consult state and federal laws to ensure that their documentation is in compliance with current guidelines.

Medicare documentation is an important and often challenging type of physical therapy documentation. We discuss Medicare documentation guidelines in Chapter 12, and we provide sample forms. In preparing this book, we discussed our framework and suggestions with many therapists and managers who have extensive experience with Medicare reimbursement. However, we caution the reader that this framework does not necessarily comply with specific Medicare requirements or standards, which change frequently. We do believe that the principles discussed in this book are applicable to all forms of documentation, including Medicare, as they are currently used in clinical settings.

We do not pretend to have invented the big ideas in this book. Indeed, we have freely borrowed the ideas of others, with the intention of putting them into a form that would be useful for students and beginning therapists. The importance of disablement models for physical therapy is a central idea, and we owe an intellectual debt to Alan Jette for his articulate writings on this subject. In 1993, Darlene Stewart and Susan Abeln wrote an extremely persuasive book entitled *Documenting Functional Outcomes in Physical Therapy*, which had an enormous impact on our thinking. These authors were among the first to propose an approach to functional outcomes documentation and to demonstrate that it can be a valuable tool for improving physical therapy practice. Marcia Hornbook Stamer's *Functional Documentation: A Process for the Physical Therapist* also helped us to develop our approach. Ken Randall and Irene McEwen's terrific article in the December 2000 issue of *Physical Therapy* on "patient-centered goals" helped us to clarify our approach to setting goals. Ginge Kettenbach's text on *Writing SOAP Notes* is a model of didactic clarity that greatly influenced our approach to writing the textbook, especially in the development of practice exercises. We found many more sources of inspiration, which are too numerous to mention here.

Finally, we do not intend that this book should be the last word on documentation in physical therapy. On the contrary, we see it as a beginning. We hope that physical therapists will continue to explore new forms of documentation that will better reflect the changing patterns of practice and that will facilitate improvements in patient care. We invite readers to send comments, suggestions, and criticisms to us and to publish alternative approaches in journals and textbooks. Discussion and debate about the best ways to document will help us to find the true path to best practice.

Lori Quinn
James Gordon

Acknowledgments

The authors would like to acknowledge the contributions by many people who provided examples, ideas, insights, and, most importantly, critiques of this book at various stages of its inception. First, we owe a debt of gratitude to current and past students of the Physical Therapy Program at New York Medical College. We have benefited so much from the thoughtful insights of students for whom this material was first designed.

Next, we would like to thank the staff and faculty of the Program in Physical Therapy at New York Medical College and the Department of Biokinesiology and Physical Therapy at the University of Southern California. Many of the faculty provided important comments for this book, wrote or reviewed case examples, or helped with editorial components.

We would also like to thank the physical therapy staff and administration at Burke Rehabilitation Hospital, White Plains, New York, for their important insights regarding documentation in the clinic. The PT staff participated in focus groups as well as ongoing discussions regarding the realities of documentation and functional outcomes.

We gratefully acknowledge the following individuals:

Stefania Bonanni
Maureen Burgess, MA, PT
Stefanie Coffey, PT
Paul Eberle, MS, PT
Anne Farrell, PhD
Robin Fillhart, MS, PT
Julie Fineman, EdM, PT
Beth Fisher, PhD, PT
Jennifer Gallaher, MS, PT
Michael Gallucci, MS, PT
Gail Harris, MS, PT
Janet Herbold, MA, PT
Kornelia Kulig, PhD, PT
Rob Landel, DPT
Cynthia Lazarra, MS, PT
Allene Mahr

Michael Majsak, EdD, PT
Agnes McConlogue, MA, PT
Dan Millrood, MS, PT
Patricia Nannariello, MS, PT
Kim O'Connor, PhD, PT
Tom Onorato, PT
Jeff Rodrigues, DPT
Mary Ruiz, MS, PT
Lisa Saladin, PT
Renee Stolove, MA, PT

We thank the many reviewers who carefully read and provided insightful comments about the book:

Nancy A. Bookstein, EdD, PT
Patricia R. Curratti, PT, MS, PCS
April Friedman, PT, MS
Rebecca Graves, MS, PT
Susan Howard, PT
David A. Lake, PT, PhD
Susan M. Roehrig, PT, PhD

We also gratefully acknowledge the work of our editors, who provided great support and encouragement during this process. Andrew Allen has contributed equal amounts of encouragement and patience, without which it is doubtful we would have seen this project through. We would also like to thank Rachel Zipperlen, Marj Fraser, and Marion Waldman, as well as the entire editorial staff, for their expert assistance in completing this project.

Last, we thank our families for their never-ending support. With gratitude:
to Eric and Annabel
to Provi, Jason, Anita, and Maddie

Lori Quinn
James Gordon

Contents

Functional Outcomes

Documentation for Rehabilitation

Theoretical Foundations

CHAPTER 1

Introduction

LEARNING OBJECTIVES

After reading this chapter and completing the exercises, the reader will be able to:

1. Identify and describe three different models of disablement.
2. Define the four levels of the Nagi model of disablement.
3. Describe the process of rehabilitation as it applies to the Nagi model.
4. Discuss the differences between the Nagi and the ICIDH-2 models of disablement.

This book outlines a method for physical therapy documentation based on the general principle that documentation should focus on *functional outcomes.* An *outcome* is a result or consequence of physical therapy intervention. A *functional outcome* is one in which the effect of treatment is on the individual's ability to accomplish a goal that is meaningful for that individual. Functional outcomes should be the focus of physical therapy documentation:

1. Examination procedures should determine relevant functional limitations and the impairments causing those limitations.
2. Goals of therapy should be explicitly defined in terms of the functional activities that the patient will be able to perform.
3. Specific interventions should be justified in terms of their effects on functional outcomes.
4. Most importantly, the success of intervention should be measured by the degree to which desired functional outcomes are achieved.

Traditional physical therapy documentation formats do not easily adapt to a functional outcomes focus. Therefore several authors have attempted to present documentation formats that are generally referred to as *functional outcomes reports* (FOR) (Stamer, 1995; Stewart, 1993). The FOR format presented in this book is based in part on ideas derived from these published documentation formats and the authors' own clinical and teaching experience.

Clearly there is no single correct way to write physical therapy documentation. Documentation must be adapted to the context in which it is written. The purpose of this book is therefore not to present a rigid format for writing documentation. Instead, the book offers a set of guidelines for writing documentation in a functional outcomes format. This set of guidelines is flexible and should be adaptable to many different practice settings. The main purpose of this book is to provide guided practice in writing functional outcomes documentation.

The framework for documentation presented herein is based on a widely accepted model of how pathologic conditions lead to disability, called the *Nagi model* (Nagi, 1965, 1991). The Nagi model is an integral part of *The Guide to Physical Therapist Practice* (2001). The main purpose of the Guide is to "help physical therapists analyze their patient/client management and describe the scope of their practice" (*The Guide to Physical Therapist Practice,* p. 12). Importantly, the Guide has helped to establish a common set of definitions and physical therapy terminology. This book attempts to use that terminology in addition to an overall conceptual framework that is consistent with that of the Guide.

Several models of the disablement process are discussed in this chapter; the Nagi model is one example. Also considered is how these models can be used to understand what physical therapists do in the diagnostic process and in planning appropriate interventions. Finally, the importance of the disability framework to documentation is discussed. The exercises at the end of the chapter provide practice in classifying conditions according to the Nagi model.

MODELS OF THE DISABLEMENT PROCESS

The use of disablement models as an organizing framework for physical therapy was one of the key conceptual developments of the 1990s (Jette, 1994). Various models of disablement have been developed and explored, including the World Health Organization (WHO) model (International Classification of Diseases, 1997), the Nagi model (Nagi, 1965), and the National Center for Medical Rehabilitation Research (NCMRR) model (National Advisory Board on Medical Rehabilitation Research, 1991). These models are illustrated in Figure 1-1. Despite differences in terminology, each model provides a framework for analyzing the various effects of acute and chronic conditions on the functioning of specific body systems, basic human performance, and people's functioning in necessary, expected, and personally desired roles in society (Jette, 1994).

The Nagi model is the basis for the documentation system proposed in this book for at least two reasons. First, as noted previously, the Guide has adopted the Nagi model. Thus this documentation model is consistent with terminology used in the Guide. Second, the Nagi model is most useful for clinical decision making. The Nagi terminology is clearly delineated and is well suited to documentation. Therefore the terminology throughout this text is based on the Nagi model.

Disablement describes the consequences of disease in terms of its effects on body functions (i.e., impairments), the ability of the individual to perform meaningful tasks (i.e., functional limitations), and the ability to fulfill one's roles in life (i.e., disability). The arrows in Figure 1-1 imply a causal chain leading from pathologic conditions to disability. Indeed, the causal links between elements in the model are useful; they help to conceptualize the relationships between findings at different levels. Nevertheless, the arrows should not be interpreted as necessarily indicating a temporal series of events. Further, the causal relations between different levels are complex and often multidirectional.

The Nagi model demonstrates that patients can be viewed from different perspectives (Figure 1-2). A therapist can describe patients' pathologic condition(s), impairments, functional limitations, or disabilities. These are not separate characteristics of the patient; they are the same characteristic, described in different measurement systems. They represent different ways of describing how a pathologic condition affects the patient and the patient's adaptation to the condition.

Disablement Models as Aids to Diagnosis

Physical therapy diagnosis is the process by which a patient's key functional limitations are identified and the causes of those functional limitations are determined. Typically the causes are stated in terms of impairments. For example, the patient's problem may be described as follows: "patient is unable to walk without assistance because of weakness in the right quadriceps and resulting inability to support weight on right leg." This diagnosis immediately suggests several possible interventions, such as strengthening exercises, orthotic and other assistive devices, and gait training. The therapist's choice of interventions depends on information about the patient's pathologic condition and other factors.

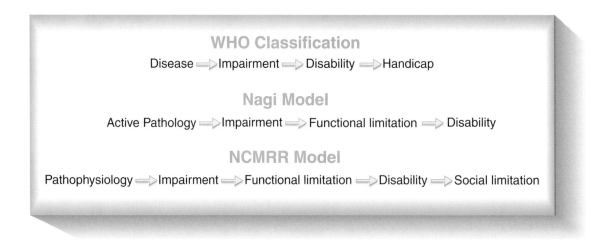

FIGURE 1-1

Different models of the disablement process.

Nagi Model

Disablement: the various impacts of pathologic conditions on the functioning of specific body systems, basic human performance, and people's functioning in necessary, expected, and personally desired roles in society.

Pathology	Impairment	Functional limitation	Disability
Damage or disruption of *cellular* processes, homeostasis, or the structural integrity of body parts	Loss or abnormality at *tissue, organ, or body system level*	Restrictions in performance at the *level of the whole person*	Inability to fulfill one's desired or necessary roles, both personal and social, at the *level of the person's relation to society*
Examples	**Examples**	**Examples**	**Examples**
• infarction of neurons in precentral gyrus of cerebral cortex • fracture of distal tibia • transtibial amputation of left leg • tear of anterior cruciate ligament of knee • viral infection of lung tissue (right lower lobe)	• paralysis of lower extremities • weakness of right biceps • impaired sensation left foot • restriction in right hip ROM • impaired proactive balance control • inadequate foot clearance during gait • poor coordination of reaching and grasping movements • inability to cough	• inability to walk on level surfaces • inability to dress oneself • inability to prepare a meal • inability to lift a carton weighing more than 30 pounds • inability to walk up and down a flight of stairs	• inability to care for oneself without assistance • inability to work at normal occupation • inability to fulfill role as spouse or parent • inability to play golf

FIGURE 1-2

The Nagi model of disablement, including clinical examples from different patient scenarios.

This example illustrates that physical therapists typically work at the interface between impairments and functional limitations. The therapist often seeks to determine which impairments are causing a patient's functional limitations. Interventions may indirectly improve function by reducing impairments, or they may directly improve function by helping the person to learn or relearn functional skills. Ideally, both types of interventions are used. The underlying pathologic condition usually is affected indirectly by physical therapy intervention; the intervention promotes healing by allowing the tissue to rest or be active at different points in the course of recovery. Occasionally the therapist attempts to directly affect tissue healing, but most often information about a patient's pathologic condition is used to help predict prognosis and time course, and these in turn will help in clinical decision making. Thus disablement models, including the Nagi model, provide an ideal framework for describing the processes of developing a diagnosis and planning appropriate intervention by the physical therapist.

TABLE 1-1 ANALYZING A PATIENT'S DISABLEMENT PROCESS USING THE NAGI MODEL	
Disablement Process	**Case Example**
DISABILITY Limitation in performance of socially defined roles and tasks within a sociocultural and physical environment	• Unable to perform social activities and volunteer work twice/week outside home
FUNCTIONAL LIMITATIONS Limitation in a performance at the level of the whole organism	• Unable to walk distances outdoors (greater than 25 ft); limited by fatigue and inability to negotiate uneven terrain • Requires physical assistance to get in and out of car
IMPAIRMENTS Anatomic, physiologic, mental or emotional abnormalities or loss	• Weakness—right hip extension, flexion, and abduction • Gait impairment—uneven stance time, uneven stride length • Limited cardiovascular endurance for walking
PATHOLOGY Interruption or interference with normal processes and efforts of the organism to regain normal state	• Right hip fracture secondary to fall in bathtub → total hip replacement (posterior approach)

Although there are causal relationships between levels in the Nagi model, these links are not obligatory. Weakness of the quadriceps muscle does not necessarily impair the ability to walk up and down stairs; an inability to walk on stairs does not necessarily prevent an individual from performing occupational activities. The crucial implication of disablement models is that a specific impairment, such as weakness, should be a focus of intervention if and only if that impairment can be demonstrated to be a causal factor in the inability to accomplish a functional activity that is necessary for the individual in his or her life activities.

Rehabilitation: The Reverse of Disablement

The Nagi model of disablement provides the conceptual framework for a "top-down approach" to understanding a patient's problems. Such an approach represents the natural way in which physical therapists solve clinical problems in a wide variety of situations. The case example in Table 1-1 provides a simplified outline of one potential disability and the levels of the disablement process for an individual who has had a total hip replacement.

Disablement models can be counterproductive if they lead to an overly reductionist approach to rehabilitation, that is, if improvements in impairments are assumed to lead to improvements in functional activities. This is a subtle example of the so-called medical model, in which it is assumed that curing a disease will automatically improve the patient's quality of life. Physical therapists fall victim to the same fallacy when they focus intervention exclusively on impairments.

This pitfall can be avoided if rehabilitation is conceptualized as the reverse and mirror image of disablement (Figure 1-3). Whereas disablement begins with a pathologic condition, rehabilitation begins with specifying the desired result in terms of the personal and social roles the patient is attempting to achieve, resume, or retain. These roles require the performance of functional skills—from self-care to household to community to occupation. The therapist must determine how these skills are limited in such ways as to prevent the fulfillment of the individual's roles. Then the therapist must ascertain why the specified functions are limited, by determining the critical neuromotor and musculoskeletal mechanisms that are impaired. These mechanisms can be considered resources that can be used in the performance of the functional skills.

Finally, the opposite of a pathologic process is *recovery*. Health is not simply the absence of disease, but an active process of healing. In many instances, especially in the acute stages, the primary goal of therapy is to promote recovery by creating an optimal environment for tissue healing and system reorganization.

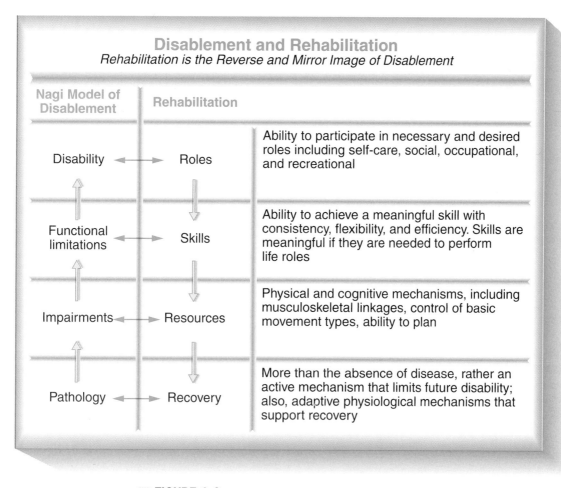

Disablement and Rehabilitation
Rehabilitation is the Reverse and Mirror Image of Disablement

Nagi Model of Disablement	Rehabilitation	
Disability	Roles	Ability to participate in necessary and desired roles including self-care, social, occupational, and recreational
Functional limitations	Skills	Ability to achieve a meaningful skill with consistency, flexibility, and efficiency. Skills are meaningful if they are needed to perform life roles
Impairments	Resources	Physical and cognitive mechanisms, including musculoskeletal linkages, control of basic movement types, ability to plan
Pathology	Recovery	More than the absence of disease, rather an active mechanism that limits future disability; also, adaptive physiological mechanisms that support recovery

FIGURE 1-3

The relationship between disablement and rehabilitation.

For example, in a patient with an acute injury to the rotator cuff musculature, the overall goal of therapy might be to prevent disability, such as the loss of a valued recreational activity. If the patient were a recreational tennis player, the ability to perform strong and accurate overhead service swings would be a functional goal. The immediate impairments would likely include pain, loss of passive range of motion, and weakness. Therapy initially would be planned to promote tissue healing by avoiding strong overhead swings and encouraging pain-free motion at the shoulder. In the post-acute stage of the rehabilitation process, therapy would be designed to increase strength and range of motion. As soon as practical and safe, the specific functional activities that are limited would be practiced. Isolated flexibility and strengthening exercises might be taught to the patient, but they would be vali-

dated by frequent retesting of the functional task. Finally, the patient would be taught proper techniques to avoid reinjury. In both acute and chronic stages, the clinical decision-making process is initiated by determining, in consultation with the patient, the personal and social roles that the patient wishes to fulfill.

The extension of the Nagi model in Figure 1-3 emphasizes that a primary goal of physical therapy is to eliminate or reduce functional limitations. Nevertheless, the emphasis on functional outcomes should not be taken to imply that it is enough to simply ignore impairments and focus exclusively on functional training and functional measures of performance. Physical therapists are trained to determine the causes of movement dysfunction, usually in terms of impairments. To ignore or neglect this aspect of physical therapy is as much a fallacy as to neglect function.

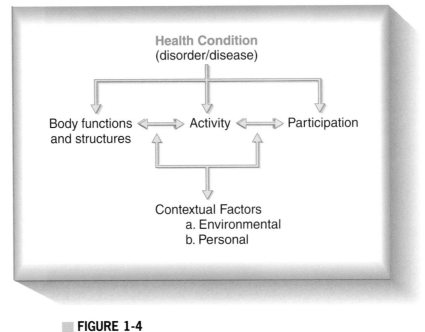

■ **FIGURE 1-4**

The ICIDH-2 model of disablement.

THE NEW WHO MODEL: ICIDH-2

In 1980 the World Health Organization (WHO) published the first version of the International Classification of Impairments, Disabilities, and Handicaps (ICIDH). This is a detailed classification system based on the disablement model presented in Figure 1-1. WHO has recently revised this classification; the revision is based on a modified disablement model (Figure 1-4).

In this new model the process of disablement is a combination of: (1) losses or abnormalities of bodily function and structure; (2) limitations of activities; and (3) restrictions in participation. Thus in at least one respect, the ICIDH-2 model clearly moves in the same directions as the extension of the Nagi model presented herein, which incorporates the process of rehabilitation as being the reverse process of disablement (see Figure 1-3). The ICIDH-2 seeks to redefine what Nagi refers to as functional limitations and disabilities in positive terms, as activity and participation. Thus, although the general structure is similar to the original WHO model, the focus of this new model is on the "positive" aspects of disablement. For example, the terms *activity* and *participation* focus on a person's abilities versus inabilities, or disabilities.

At the same time the revised ICIDH model relinquishes the notion of simple, unidirectional causal links between levels. As seen in Figure 1-4, the individual's pathologic state (health condition) becomes a broader category that influences all other levels. Furthermore, contextual factors, both extrinsic (environmental) and intrinsic (personal), are specifically identified as affecting the relationship between impairments and activities, and activities and participation. Personal factors can consist of such things as family support, whereas extrinsic factors might include environmental barriers. These are important additions that highlight the multiple factors that can be related to any one person's "disability."

The differences among the various disablement models represent more than simply differences in terminology; important theoretical differences also exist (which are beyond the scope of this book). Nevertheless, these differences are small compared with the overwhelming similarity of the models. All are based on the assumption that the process of disablement can be analyzed at multiple levels. In the 1990s the Nagi model gained considerable acceptance in North America, whereas the WHO model has been used more widely in Europe, Australia, and Asia. It will be interesting to observe whether the new ICIDH-2 model will unify the world's terminology over the next decade.

TABLE 1-2 CLASSIFICATION USING THE NAGI DISABLEMENT MODEL		
Nagi Model of Disablement	**Organization Level**	**Level of Measurement**
Disability	Whole person in relation to society	Participation/level of assistance/quality of life
Functional limitations	Whole person	Performance/skill (Goal attainment)
Impairments	Body organ or body system	Functions of specific body systems
Pathology	Tissue or cellular	Medical diagnosis

FUNCTIONAL OUTCOMES: MORE THAN SIMPLY A DOCUMENTATION STRATEGY

The organizing principles chosen by the therapist for documentation illustrate the organizing principles chosen for diagnosis and treatment. Similarly, a haphazard approach to documentation is likely to reflect a haphazard approach to physical therapy evaluation and intervention. Therefore the organizational framework for documentation presented in this book represents more than simply a way to organize notes. The method of documentation is based on two assumptions: (1) a primary purpose of physical therapy evaluation is to define the specific functional outcomes that need to be achieved, and (2) the criterion for judging the effectiveness of treatment should be whether those outcomes are achieved.

In other words, if it is accepted that physical therapy documentation should be focused on functional outcomes, then logically, physical therapy evaluation and intervention should be focused on functional outcomes. Neither the format presented here nor any FOR format should be viewed as simply a *post hoc* method for justifying reimbursement of physical therapy services in the managed care environment. Continuing to view the role of physical therapists as treating impairments while recasting what they do as functionally based "in order to satisfy third-party payers" makes no sense. The purpose of FOR documentation is to provide an explicit and prospective framework by which physical therapists can (1) analyze the reasons for disablement in their patients, (2) formulate strategies for preventing or reversing that disablement, and (3) explain and justify the resulting clinical decisions they make.

CLASSIFICATION ACCORDING TO THE DISABLEMENT MODEL

Writing documentation requires the physical therapist to develop skill in classifying the various aspects of the patient's condition using the Nagi model as a framework. The classification has two bases: the organizational level at which function is observed, and the level of measurement (Table 1-2).

For example, the observation that a patient has an infection of the femur (osteomyelitis) is an example of pathologic information (at the tissue level; a medical diagnosis). The medical diagnosis usually includes the nature of the pathology (e.g., infection, tumor), its location, and the timing relative to onset (i.e., acute vs. chronic). Weakness of the quadriceps muscle is reduced function of a body system (muscular); thus it is an impairment. It is measured in the frame of reference defined by the body system's function. The muscular system is defined by its ability to produce force over time. Weakness is measured in terms of the force output possible in a defined set of conditions.

An inability to walk is defined as a functional limitation because it is a deficit in the ability of the whole person to successfully perform an activity. Functional limitations are measured in terms of performance or skill. Considering whether, and to what degree, the goal of the action has been attained, is most useful. A patient's inability to care for his or her child would be a disability. It is measured at the level of the individual's social interaction, which can be quantified along three dimensions: (1) participation in desired or expected social roles, (2) the level of assistance required to achieve that participation, and (3) quality of life. Exercise 1-1 at the end of this chapter provides an opportunity to practice classifying various statements within the Nagi framework.

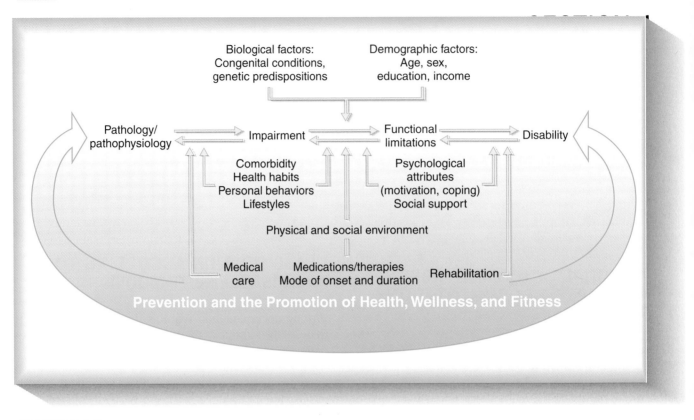

Biological factors:
Congenital conditions,
genetic predispositions

Demographic factors:
Age, sex,
education, income

Pathology/
pathophysiology → Impairment → Functional
limitations → Disability

Comorbidity
Health habits
Personal behaviors
Lifestyles

Psychological
attributes
(motivation, coping)
Social support

Physical and social environment

Medical
care

Medications/therapies
Mode of onset and duration

Rehabilitation

Prevention and the Promotion of Health, Wellness, and Fitness

FIGURE 1-5

An expanded disablement model reprinted with permission from the *Guide to Physical Therapist Practice (2001)*. This model highlights the importance of prevention as a component of physical therapy practice.

PREVENTION AND HEALTH PROMOTION

Primary, secondary, and tertiary prevention are important aspects of physical therapy practice and are within the scope of physical therapist practice (*Guide to Physical Therapist Practice*, 2001) (see Figure 1-5). The purpose of prevention in physical therapy is to "prevent impairments, functional limitation, or disabilities by identifying disablement risk factors during the diagnostic process and by buffering the disablement process" (*Guide to Physical Therapist Practice*, 2001, p S24).

For documentation purposes, physical therapists must clearly document specific risk factors, the relationships between those risk factors, and the functional limitations or disabilities that might result if the risk factors are not addressed. For example, if a patient presents with risk factors for osteoporosis (e.g., female, low bone density, history of wrist fracture, decreased lumbar spine range of motion), then each of these should be documented in their appropriate section of the evaluation report. In the Assessment section (see Chapter 8), the therapist would then discuss the relationship of these factors to the risk of osteoporosis and then justify the need for physical therapy intervention as a means to decrease this risk.

In this book, prevention is discussed as it is appropriate to each of the chapters. For further information on prevention in physical therapy, see the *Guide to Physical Therapist Practice*, specifically Preferred Practice Patterns 4A, 5A, 6A, and 7A.

SUMMARY

- This chapter has presented a conceptual framework for a specific documentation strategy organized around functional outcomes.

- Functional outcomes should be the focus of physical therapy documentation; this involves documenting functional limitations, setting functional goals, justifying interventions, and measuring their success based on the effects on functional outcomes.

- Disablement describes the consequences of disease in terms of its effects on body functions (i.e., impairments), the ability of the individual to perform meaningful tasks (i.e., functional limitations), and the ability to fulfill one's roles in life (i.e., disability).

- There are many different disablement models; this book follows terminology used in the Nagi model: disability, functional limitations, impairments, and pathology.

- Physical therapists typically work at the interface between impairments and functional limitations.

- Rehabilitation is the reverse of disablement. Whereas disablement begins with pathology, rehabilitation begins with specifying the desired end result in terms of the personal and social roles that the patient is attempting to achieve, resume, or retain.

- The next chapters offer a set of guidelines for writing documentation in a functional outcomes format, which should be adaptable to many different practice settings.

EXERCISE 1-1

Classify each statement according to which level of the Nagi model it reflects: pathologic condition (P), impairment (I), functional limitation (F), or disability (D). Statements may reflect positive attributes (e.g., recovery, resources, skills, or roles).

Statement	Classification
1. Patient has 0° to 120° of active abduction left shoulder.	F
2. Patient can walk up to 50 feet on level surfaces indoors.	F
3. Partial tear of right anterior cruciate ligament.	P
4. Patient is unable to work at previous occupation of a salesperson.	D
5. Strength right knee flexion 3/5 on manual muscle test.	I
6. Patient needs minimal assistance to dress lower body.	F
7. Transfemoral amputation of right lower extremity.	P
8. Heart rate increases from 80 beats per minute to 140 after climbing 1 flight of stairs.	I
9. Patient was diagnosed with multiple sclerosis 10/1/98.	P
10. Patient is able to eat soup from a bowl independently.	D
11. Left lateral pinch strength 15 lbs.	I
12. Patient transfers from bed to wheelchair independently with use of a sliding board.	F
13. Patient has full passive range of motion in left knee.	I
14. Patient is able to reach for and grasp a cup located at shoulder height.	F
15. Patient can stand at kitchen sink for 2 minutes.	D
16. Patient is unable to perform a straight leg raise.	I

Continued

Statement	Classification
17. Patient has pain in right shoulder, 5/10 on Visual Analog Scale, whenever he raises his arm above shoulder height.	I
18. Patient has a personal aide for 4 hours per day to assist with daily care and household chores.	D
19. Patient is unable to cook using the stove, and needs moderate assistance to prepare all meals.	F
20. Patient is able to transfer from floor to her wheelchair within 2 minutes.	F
21. Patient was diagnosed with T8 spinal cord injury after motor vehicle accident in 1999.	P
22. Patient is able to enter most buildings in his wheelchair, provided an appropriate ramp is present.	F
23. Partial rotator cuff tear of right shoulder.	P
24. Patient is able to return to modified work duty as a bus driver.	D
25. Patient can walk up to 300 feet in the hospital corridor with minimal assistance and walker.	F

CHAPTER 2

Essentials of Documentation

LEARNING OBJECTIVES

After reading this chapter and completing the exercises, the reader will be able to:

1. Discuss the history of the medical record and documentation.
2. Identify the four basic types of physical therapy notes.
3. Discuss the pros and cons of different documentation formats.
4. List the different purposes that documentation serves.
5. Use the correct method for signing notes and correcting errors in documentation.
6. Use people-first language in all forms of communication.
7. Appropriately use and interpret common rehabilitation and medical abbreviations.

DOCUMENTATION: AN OVERVIEW

Physical therapists (PTs) and physical therapist assistants (PTAs) often view documentation as an onerous chore. At best, it is considered a necessary evil, to be accomplished as quickly and painlessly as possible. At worst, it is a conspiracy by bureaucrats to waste therapists' time and limit patient access to essential services. Despite this view, the modern medical record is one of the most important achievements in the development of twentieth century medicine. At the beginning of the twentieth century, the notion of a patient-centered chart that stayed with the patient was almost unheard of. Instead, records were kept by individual practitioners, and often the records were haphazard. The development of a comprehensive patient-centered chart, professionally written and clearly organized, enabled direct improvements in patient care by promoting accurate and timely communication among professionals. It also allowed improvements in patient care indirectly by facilitating better review of the process. The medical chart is the collector and organizer of the primary data for clinical research. It is also an essential teaching device. Students and novice clinicians learn about how to provide patient care by reading the documentation written by expert clinicians. It is doubtful that health care would have reached the present level of accomplishment without the changes in documentation over the past century. Moreover, future improvements in patient care will be associated with, and enabled by, changes in the way the process is documented. Documentation is therefore a dynamic phenomenon, ever changing. The dominant formats can be expected to adapt to the changes in health care.

Of course, changes in health care have occurred not just in the clinical domain, but also in the economic and social domains. The United States is in the midst of a period in which fundamental changes are occurring in the way in which health care is financed and compensated. Third-party payers, often organized as health maintenance organizations, are moving away from reimbursing procedures and toward reimbursing outcomes. In other words, practitioners must clearly justify the treatment they are implementing in terms of the outcomes that will be achieved.

Despite its importance, documentation is often viewed negatively by therapists for at least two reasons. First, and most obvious, too little time is dedicated to documentation in the clinic. Second, therapists are given relatively little training in documentation. When proper guidelines and adequate training are provided, appropriate outcomes-based documentation does not have to be extremely labor-intensive. However, documentation is a skill that should be valued by therapists, educators, and supervisors, similar to any other physical therapy skill. Thus students and therapists must spend dedicated, focused time to learn the "skill" of documentation. Skill develops with practice, practice, and more practice.

Skill in documentation is the hallmark of a professional approach to therapy and is one of the characteristics that distinguishes a professional from a technician. Therapists should take pride in their professional writing; it is the window through which they are judged by other professionals. In fact, it could be argued that documentation of services rendered is just as important as the actual rendering of the services. Supervisors must recognize that good documentation takes time, and therapists must be provided with that time.

In this chapter, some of the essential aspects of documentation are now addressed. Different classifications and formats for physical therapy documentation are presented, as well as critical aspects of information that should be included and the manner in which it should be reported.

TYPES OF NOTES

Four basic types of medical record documentation exist: the initial evaluation, daily or per session notes, reexamination or progress notes, and the discharge summary. These are described in detail in the American Physical Therapy Association (APTA) *Guidelines for Physical Therapy Documentation* (Appendix A; APTA, 2001). Some of the key features of each type are described in the following text.

Initial Evaluation (Written by Physical Therapist)

- Required at onset of episode of PT care
- Documents impairments and functional limitations
- Identifies diagnosis, or cause of functional limitations
- Sets goals along with anticipated timeline
- Specifies a plan of care that directly addresses the problems and will be likely to achieve the goals

Daily or Per Session Notes (Written by Physical Therapist or Physical Therapist Assistant)

- Required for every visit encounter
- States what the PT or PTA and patient have done, and why
- Reports changes in patient/client status

Reexamination or Progress Notes (Written by Physical Therapist)

- Provides an update of patient/client status over a number of visits or certain period of time
- Restates the goals
- States what the therapist and patient have done, and why
- Details effectiveness of intervention in achieving the goals, and when indicated, revision of the goals and plan of care
- States how much longer physical therapy intervention is indicated, and provides justification for continued services

Discharge Summary (Written by Physical Therapist)

- Specifies criteria or reasons for discharge
- Summarizes effectiveness of intervention in changing initial problem and meeting expected goals
- Outlines relevant recommendations for future

The main aspects of this book focus on documentation of the initial evaluation components. Special considerations for writing daily or per session notes and the reexamination (progress notes) are specifically covered in Chapter 11. Documentation of discharge summary and other types of documentation are discussed in Chapter 12. Additional readings on different types of physical therapy documentation are available in Stewart and Abeln (1993) and Stamer (1995).

DOCUMENTATION FORMATS

Many possible formats can be used for writing notes. Sometimes a facility or institution mandates a particular format. More often, usage of a particular format is not officially required but is instead established by tradition and the desire for consistency. In these cases, PTs, PTAs, and students should use the format in general use within the institution. A particular format does not guarantee well-written documentation; it just makes the process easier. The principles of well-written documentation can be applied in any format.

Narrative Format

The simplest form of documentation recounts what happened in a therapist-patient encounter. In this format, therapists can, and should, develop their own outline of information to cover. These outlines can be more or less detailed. The specific information listed in each heading is left to the writer's discretion, although some facilities provide guidelines for what should be covered under each heading. Nevertheless, the writer is prone to omissions with this type of format. With a narrative format, the lack of structure and sub-headings leads to a high degree of variability (both within and between different writers). Furthermore, if information is not included, it is assumed it was not tested, whereas the writer may have inadvertently omitted the testing information. In even moderately complex cases, the narrative format can sometimes be unwieldy and difficult to read.

SOAP Format

The SOAP note is a highly structured documentation format. It was developed in the 1960s at the University of Vermont by Dr. Lawrence Weed as part of the problem-oriented medical record (POMR). In this type of medical record, each patient chart was headed by a numbered list of patient problems (usually developed by the primary physician). When entering documentation, each professional would refer to the number of the problem he or she was writing about, and then write a note using SOAP format. The SOAP format requires the practitioner to enter information in the order of the acronym's initials: *Subjective-Objective-Assessment-Plan* (see Chapter 11 for more detailed information on writing SOAP notes).

The POMR was not widely adopted, perhaps because it was ahead of its time. Interestingly, however, the SOAP format did catch on and is now widely used by different professionals, despite the fact that it is no longer connected to its parent concept, the POMR. A major advantage of the SOAP format is its widespread acceptance and the resulting familiarity with the format. On the plus side, it emphasizes clear, complete, and well-organized reporting of findings with a natural progression from data collection to assessment to plan. On the other hand, it has generally been associated with an overly brief and concise style, including extensive use of abbreviations and acronyms, a style that is often difficult for nonprofessionals to interpret. On a more substantive note, Delitto and Snyder-Mackler

(1995) have commented that the SOAP format encourages a sequential rather than integrative approach to clinical decision making by promoting a tendency to simply collect all possible data before assessing it. From the PT's perspective, the principal difficulty with the SOAP note is the lack of emphasis on functional outcomes. However, the SOAP note can be adapted to reflect functional outcomes and thus can provide a useful framework for documenting daily notes and progress notes (see Chapter 11).

Functional Outcome Report Format

The functional outcome report (FOR) format is a relatively new documentation format. It was developed in the 1990s as changes in the economics of health care led to increased emphasis on functional outcomes. The FOR format focuses on documenting the ability to perform meaningful functional activities rather than isolated musculoskeletal, neuromuscular, cardiopulmonary, or integumentary impairments. When the format is implemented properly, FOR documentation establishes the rationale for therapy by indicating the links between such impairments and the disability they cause in the patient. FOR documentation also emphasizes readability by health care personnel not familiar with PT jargon (at the expense of increased time to write the documentation). More important, it promotes a style of clinical decision making (PT diagnosis) that begins with the functional problems and assesses the specific impairments that cause the functional limitations.

Several authors have presented frameworks for FOR documentation. The most well-developed and structured format is that of Stewart and Abeln (1993). Their book and articles have played a major role in promoting the idea that documentation should be focused on functional outcomes, and many of their ideas have been adapted in developing the format presented in this book. Their format was not adopted for this text for two reasons. First, the format is too highly structured and difficult to adapt to different clinical contexts. Second, their book and format are entirely focused on orthopedic physical therapy and thus translation into other contexts is difficult. Nevertheless, this book is highly recommended especially because of its strong emphasis on the need for FOR documentation. It also contains excellent examples of effective letters to insurance companies.

Another format for functional outcomes documentation is described by Stamer (1995), who proposed a modified SOAP format incorporating functional documentation. In addition, in her text on SOAP documentation for PTs and PTAs, Kettenbach (1995) describes alternate approaches in each section for making the format more focused on functional outcomes.

WHAT CONSTITUTES "DOCUMENTATION"?

The APTA *Guidelines for Physical Therapy Documentation* state that documentation is "any entry into the client record, such as consultation report, initial examination report, progress note, flow sheet/checklist that identifies the care/service provided, reexamination or summation of care" (see Appendix A). It encompasses the preparation and assembly of records to authenticate and communicate the care given by a health care provider and the reasons for giving that care.

Documentation takes many forms, including the following:

- Written reports
- Standardized forms
- Charts and graphs
- Drawings
- Photographs
- Videotapes, audiotapes
- Physical specimens

The importance of use of other forms of documentation aside from straight narrative notes cannot be overemphasized. Figure 2-1 provides an example of a graph that is used to chart a patient's progress. Providing a visualization of the patient's progress provides tremendous value for the reader. The saying "a picture is worth a thousand words" is very applicable. Furthermore, simple charts and graphs can improve readability and readily focus a reader on the critical issues.

Figure 2-2 provides detailed information in an easy-to-read format.

USE OF STANDARDIZED ASSESSMENT TOOLS

The use of standardized assessment tools is an integral part of PT documentation. However, standardized tools are designed for a variety of purposes. Therapists must consider the purpose and design of the tool before using it for evaluative purposes. This book focuses on those tools that may be used to assess change over time (evaluative) and those that are useful in objectively or quantitatively describing impairments or functional skills. However, using standardized tools often is important for other reasons, such as to discriminate the need for services or predict risk for certain problems.

The therapist must have knowledge of the reliability and validity of an evaluation tool and understand the purpose for which the tool was designed to use it properly. Part III of the *Guide to Physical Therapist Practice* was recently developed as a resource on standardized tests and measures. Literally hundreds of evaluation tools are summarized in this document, including information on where to obtain these tools. Part III of *The Guide* is available on CD-ROM through the APTA. Chapters 5, 6, and 7 provide tables with information on commonly used assessment tools that measure primarily at the level of disability, function, and impairment, respectively.

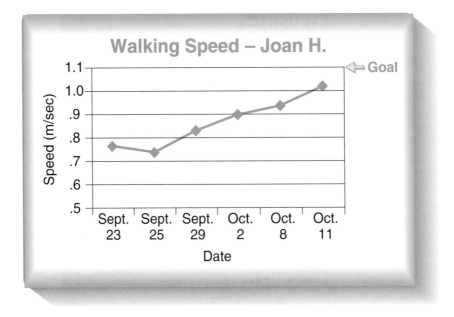

FIGURE 2-1

Graphs can be very useful in providing a visualization of patient progress.

Functional skills	Level of A	Comments
Rolling in bed	Ind.	
Positioning in bed	Min A	Needs verbal cues to use L UE and L LE to assist in movement
Supine → sitting in bed	Mod A to R Sup. to L	Can bring legs over side of bed to R, unable to use L arm and trunk to push up to sit
Sitting → supine in bed	Ind.	
Transfer bed to wheelchair	Min A c̄ sliding board	Needs A for proper set up and to initiate movement

A

Muscle Group	Strength (MMT)	
	Right	Left
Knee extension	3+/5	5/5
Knee flexion	3+/5	4/5
Ankle dorsiflexion	4/5	4/5
Ankle plantarflexion	4/5	5/5

B

FIGURE 2-2

A and **B,** Tables can provide detailed information in an easy-to-read format.

CRITICAL ASPECTS OF NOTEWRITING

PT documentation serves many purposes. These include the following:

Communication with Other Professionals

- Ensures coordination and continuity of patient care
- Organizes the planning of treatment strategies

Clinical Decision Making

- Explains treatment rationale

Legal Record of PT Management of Patient

- Specifies that patient has been seen and that intervention has occurred
- Serves as a business record
- Is often used to determine how much should be billed for a visit

Examples of Uses by Others

- Make decisions about reimbursement
- Decide discharge and future placement
- Is used as a quality assurance tool
- Is used as data for research on outcomes

LEGAL ASPECTS OF NOTEWRITING

Documentation in a medical record is a legal document. Therapists should treat notewriting very seriously and understand that their notes may be scrutinized not only for payment of services but also for legal reasons.

The Centers for Medicare and Medicaid Services (CMS; formally known as HCFA) provides recommended guidelines for documentation purposes related to patients who receive Medicare or Medicaid. Because these guidelines are updated frequently, readers are referred to the HCFA website (www.cms.gov) for the most up-to-date information. Readers are also referred to APTA *Guidelines for Physical Therapy Documentation* (Appendix A) and Scott (2000) for more detailed information on legal aspects of documentation.

Several key legal aspects pertinent to physical therapy documentation are outlined below.

- Handwritten entries should be legible and written in ink.
- All notes must be dated with the date that the note was written. Backdating is illegal and should never be done. If a note is not written on the date that treatment or an evaluation is performed, that information should be included in the note. Current CMS guidelines also recommend indicating the time the note was written (for notes in an interdisciplinary medical record).
- All notes must be signed, followed by the writer's professional abbreviation. The APTA House of Delegates (APTA HOD, 1999) has recommended use of a standard abbreviation, PT, for physical therapists, PTA for physical therapist assistants, SPT for student physical therapist, and SPTA for student physical therapist assistant. These abbreviations must follow all signatures.
- SPTs or SPTAs (those individuals who are enrolled in a PT or PTA educational program) are allowed to write notes in the medical record. These notes must be signed and dated by the student and also must be co-signed by a supervising licensed PT or PTA (refer to APTA Guidelines, Appendix A).
- If an error is made, the therapist should place a single line through the erroneous word, and write his or her initials near the crossed-out word. The date and time of correction should also be included.
- Blank lines or large empty spaces should be avoided in the record. A single straight line should be drawn through any open spaces in a report.
- The writer should use only those abbreviations authorized by his or her facility (Appendix B provides a list of commonly used abbreviations in rehabilitation settings).
- Informed consent should be documented. The patient/client should be asked to acknowledge understanding and consent before intervention is initiated. Many facilities have a separate form for this purpose.

Sometimes conflicts or personal issues arise between therapists and patients, and between patients and their physicians or other medical professionals. Generally, conflicts of this nature should not be included in documentation. Only information that is directly relevant to the patient's medical condition, prognosis, or intervention plan should be documented.

AVOIDING LABELS AND DEROGATORY STATEMENTS

People-first language should be used in all forms of documentation and communication. The 1991 APTA HOD Resolution 06-91-25-34 (Program 50) states that "physical therapy practitioners have an obligation to provide non-judgmental care to all persons who need it. They should be guided in their written and spoken communication by the Guidelines for Reporting and Writing About People with Disabilities." (The *Guidelines for Reporting and Writing About People With Disabilities* [1996] are printed in a brochure, available through the University of Kansas.) For example, a patient should not be described as "a T12 para," but rather "a man with T12-level paraplegia." Other inappropriate examples are "amputees," "stroke victims," and even "cerebral palsy child." Furthermore, labeling patients with such terms as *confused, agitated,* or *noncompliant,* for example, focuses the reader on the label rather than the person, and the two become invariably linked. Rather, specific behaviors of a patient should be described. Simply because a patient may not be performing a home exercise program, he or she should not be identified as a "noncompliant patient." Instead, the patient might be described as "a patient, man, or woman" and at some later point in the documentation, it should be noted that he or she "has not consistently complied with the home program."

Therapists should also be careful to avoid derogatory statements about patients. Such terms as "Pt. complains…" or "Pt. suffers from…" have negative connotations and should be avoided. Rather, "Pt. reports…" or "Pt. has a diagnosis of…" reflect more objective statements.

CONCISENESS IN WRITING AND USE OF ABBREVIATIONS

Writing a medical record has some specific characteristics that differentiate it from traditional narrative writing. For example, medical documentation should be appropriately concise. Time is often limited in health care settings; thus wordiness and undue lengthiness should be minimized. One way to save time in medical documentation is by not using full sentence structures and using abbreviations. For example, rather than stating "The patient can walk in the hospital corridor for 50 feet with minimal assistance," it can be shortened to "Pt. walks in hospital corridor 50′ c̄ min A." Eliminating words such as "the," "for," "an," or "a" can

significantly reduce wordiness and improve readability of a medical note.

The first question that must be addressed regarding use of abbreviations is "Who will be the reader of this note?" If the answer is "another physical therapist or physical therapist assistant (and no other person)," therapists can freely use abbreviations and appropriate PT terminology. However, if only a slight possibility exists that the note might be read by another professional (e.g., physician or nurse) or by a nonprofessional (e.g., administrative staff, claims auditor, member of a jury), uncommon abbreviations and jargon almost certainly will impede understanding. Furthermore, if the writer is in doubt about the use of an abbreviation, it is best to spell out the word. The time saved writing an abbreviation may not be worth it if it cannot be interpreted by anyone else.

Clearly, common medical abbreviations can be useful time-saving devices. Appendix B provides a list of commonly accepted medical abbreviations that can be used for PT documentation in a medical chart. Although this list is not all encompassing, it represents abbreviations that are most likely to be understood by a range of medical professionals. Several books provide a more comprehensive listing of all types of medical abbreviations (Davis, 2001; Skalko, 1998). Furthermore, hospitals and health care facilities often develop their own list of abbreviations that are considered acceptable in that institution, and those lists are likely to be more encompassing than those listed here. PTs and PTAs should follow those guidelines set by individual institutions

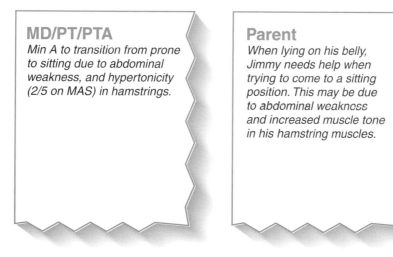

MD/PT/PTA
Min A to transition from prone to sitting due to abdominal weakness, and hypertonicity (2/5 on MAS) in hamstrings.

Parent
When lying on his belly, Jimmy needs help when trying to come to a sitting position. This may be due to abdominal weakness and increased muscle tone in his hamstring muscles.

FIGURE 2-3

Notewriting is audience specific. This figure shows two different wordings for documenting transitional skills in a young child with cerebral palsy. When a note will be read primarily by a parent or professional who is not familiar with common medical terminology, terms should be defined in an understandable and meaningful way.

when considering the appropriateness of specific abbreviations.

Documentation that is sent to insurance companies, and particularly to patients or their families, should make more limited use of jargon and abbreviations (Figure 2-3). If uncommon medical terminology is used, it should be defined in laymen's terms. This practice is critical in such areas as developmental assessments for young children because parents and educators are often the primary readers of the reports. Providing definitions for ambiguous terminology is essential to improving the reader's understanding of the report.

The *best* way to write clear, concise notes quickly is to avoid unnecessary and irrelevant facts and conclusions. Merely because the therapist has observed something does not make it appropriate to include in the note. The note should include only those observations and interpretations that are essential for documenting the patient's condition. Omitting nonessential items makes the note more readable and more efficient to write.

THE AUDIENCE

The overuse of abbreviations and jargon is a symptom of a more serious problem: the use of a private language in which much of the rationale for treatment is left implicit. If it is assumed that the reader of a note is among the *cognoscenti,* in which he or she must be able to decipher the abbreviations and strange terms, then why bother explaining what was done and why? Too often it seems as if such a philosophy guides the writing of notes. The critical elements of the clinical reasoning process cannot be omitted with the assumption that the reader will "fill in the blanks." The therapist has a professional responsibility to explain what has been done and what will be done, and why, in clear, unambiguous terms that will be understandable to all those authorized to read a therapist's notes.

Certain types of documentation are intended for the primary readership of the patient. For example, a home exercise program should be written in lay terminology, avoiding abbreviations and unclear terminology. Another example is note writing in pediatric practice, in which developmental evaluations are read primarily by parents and service coordinators. In this situation, terminology should be clarified but not excluded altogether. Professional notes should not be written in purely lay terminology. However, documentation can be written in such as way as to be readable by those outside the profession.

SUMMARY

Good documentation is primarily a matter of establishing good habits. Chief among these is timeliness: writing notes at the time of an examination or intervention. In addition, physical therapists must always consider the legal status of their documentation. Finally, therapists must ask whether their notes, if referred to at a later date, would clearly establish what was done and why.

In summary, documentation should fulfill the following criteria:

- Timeliness

  Written as close as possible to the time of the evaluation or intervention

  All notes accurately dated (no backdating)

- Legibility

- Understandability

  Avoidance of jargon

- Conciseness

  Excess verbiage avoided

  Accepted abbreviations used

- Quantitative

  Use of numbers whenever possible

- Authenticity

  No editing of prior notes

  Crossing out mistakes with a single line and initial/date

  Writing your own notes

- Courtesy

  No argument with or disparagement of other professionals

  No expression of personal feelings toward patient

  Use of people-first language

- Confidentiality

  No discussion of patient with others not directly involved in treatment

- Completeness

  No blank lines

  All forms completed

  Every note and page signed and dated with appropriate abbreviation (PT, PTA, SPT, SPTA; students require countersignature)

EXERCISE 2-1

PEOPLE-FIRST LANGUAGE

Therapists should avoid "labeling" patients and should always use people-first language in both oral and written communication. For each of the phrases below, decide first whether the phrase is appropriate. If it is, write "appropriate" in the space provided. If it is not, rewrite the phrase so that it reflects person-first language or restructure the sentence to provide a more objective or positive description of the patient (much of this exercise and the answers are adapted or reprinted with permission from Martin, 1999).

1. A quadriplegic will require help with transfers.

   A pt c̄ C-2 level quadriplegic will require A c̄ transfers

2. The patient was afflicted with multiple sclerosis when she was in her 20s.

   appropriate

3. Many PTs are involved in foot clinics for diabetics.

   appropriate

4. Have you finished the documentation for that shoulder in room 316?

5. The patient complained of pain in the right upper extremity.

   Pt. reported pain in R UE

6. A care plan for a total knee patient typically involves a strong element of patient education.

   appropriate

7. Although this computer program was designed for the disabled, able-bodied users will also find it helpful.

8. Because of a spinal cord injury, the patient was confined to a wheelchair.

   appropriate

9. Nine of 10 patients receiving physical therapy expressed interest in a group exercise session.

   appropriate

10. The patient is behaving like a child.

11. Which therapist is treating the brain-injured patient in room 216?

12. The stroke victim can often return to work.

13. The patient refused to modify her footwear choice even after the therapist told her not wear 2-inch heels.

    appropriate

14. I'll put my 10:00 on the machine while my 10:15 gets a hot pack.

15. The patient suffers from Parkinson's disease.

    appropriate

EXERCISE 2-2

INTERPRETING ABBREVIATIONS

For the each of the following statements, write the entire statement, interpreting the abbreviations.

EXAMPLE: Pt. is I in all ADLs
  Patient is independent in all activities of daily living.

1. MMT 3/5 R quads
   manual muscle test 3/5ths Right quadriceps

2. Pt. can stand s̄ A for 30 sec s̄ LOB
   Patient can stand assistance for 30 seconds

3. Pt. can transfer bed → w/c c̄ mod A using SB
   Patient can transfer to bed from wheelchair with moderate Assistance using

4. Pt. instructed in performing R SAQ, 3 sets × 10 reps
   Patient instructed in performing R

5. PROM R ankle DF 5°
   Passive range of motion Right ankle 5 degrees of freedom

6. Received Rx from MD for WBAT on L LE
   Received prescription from doctor for water bath on left lower extremity

7. Pt. instructed to perform HEP b.i.d., 10 reps each ex
   Patient instructed to preform twice a day 10 repetitions for each exercise

8. Pt. admitted to ER 10/12/00 with GCS of 4
   Patient admitted into Emergency Room 10/12/00 with

9. Medical dx: R hip fracture c̄ ORIF
   Medical diagnosis: Right hip fracture with open reduction internal fixation

10. AROM B LEs WFL
    Active range of motion lower extremities

11. Pt. instructed in use of TENS unit, on prn basis
    Patient instructed in use of transcutaneous electrical nerve stimulation unit on an as needed basis

12. CPT performed for 20 min; P&V RLL
    Chest physical therapy performed for 20 min. Right Lower lobe

13. Pt. was d/c'd from NICU on 3/3/00
    Patient was discharged from neonatal intensive care unit on 3/3/00.

14. PMH: IDDM × 5 yrs, HBP × 10 yrs
    Prior medical history: Insulin Dependent Diabetes melatus at 5yrs old and high blood pressure at 10yrs old.

15. MRI revealed mod L MCA CVA
    Magnetic resonance imaging revealed Moderate left Cerebrovascular Accident.

EXERCISE 2-3

CONCISE DOCUMENTATION AND USE OF ABBREVIATIONS

Rewrite these notes as if you were writing them in a medical record. Consider condensing sentence structure, such as eliminating unnecessary words. Use abbreviations whenever possible.

EXAMPLE: Patient can walk a distance of 50 feet in the hospital corridors.
   Pt. walks 50 ft in hospital corridors.

1. Patient underwent a procedure called a coronary artery bypass graft on 3/17/99.

   Pt. underwent CABG on 3/17/99.

2. Therapist will coordinate practice of activities of daily living with occupational therapist and with nursing staff.

   PT coordinate practice of ADL c̄ OT and nursing staff.

3. The patient's heart rate changed from 90 to 120 beats per minute after 3 minutes of walking at a comfortable speed.

   Pt.'s HR ↑ from 90bpm to 120bpm after 3min. of walking at a comfortable speed.

4. The patient's obstetric/gynecologic doctor reported that this patient has been experiencing low back pain throughout her pregnancy.

   Pt.'s OBGYN reported this Pt. experienced LBP throughout pregnancy

5. Patient's daughter reports that patient has had a recent decrease in her functional abilities and has a history of falls.

   Pt.'s daughter reports Pt. had recent ↓ in functional abilities and Hx of falls.

6. The patient's breath sounds were decreased bilaterally. The patient was instructed in performing deep breathing exercises twice per day.

   Pt.'s breath sounds ↓ bilat.   Pt. instructed to preform DBE b.id.

7. Patient's wife reports that the patient has had a history of chronic low back pain for the past 15 years.

   Pt.'s wife reports Pt. has Hx of Chronic LBP for past 15 yrs.

8. The patient's long-term goal is to be able to walk using only a straight cane.

   Pt.'s LTG is to walk using a straight cane.

9. Deep tendon reflex of right biceps was recorded as a 2+.

   DTR of R biceps was a 2+

10. Patient can ascend and descend 1 flight of stairs independently, using 1 hand on railing.

    Pt. can go ↑ and ↓ 1 fligh of stairs I, using 1 hand on railing.

11. Prescription received for physical therapy to include therapeutic exercise and gait training.

    Rx for PT to include TE and GT

12. Resident is 82 years old and has a primary medical diagnosis of congestive heart failure.

    82 yrs old Pt c̄ PMD of CHF.

13. Electrocardiogram revealed ventricular tachycardia.

    EKG revealed V tachycardia.

14. Patient suffered a cerebrovascular accident, with resultant hemiplegia of the right upper and lower extremity.

    Pt. suffered CVA c̄ resultant hemiplegia of R UE and LE.

15. The home health aide was instructed in assisting patient to perform active-assistive range of motion exercises, including straight leg raises and hip abduction in supine.

    HHA instructed in A Pt. c̄ AAROM ex, Including Straight leg raises and hip abd. in supine

Overview of Functional Outcomes Approach to Documentation: The Initial Evaluation Format

LEARNING OBJECTIVES

After reading this chapter and completing the exercises at the end, the reader will be able to:

1. Outline a model for organizing an initial evaluation based on a functional outcomes approach.
2. Identify the basic elements for each of the six sections of the initial evaluation format.
3. Describe the relationship between *The Guide's* patient/client management model and the six sections of the initial evaluation format.
4. Categorize components of an initial evaluation into the initial evaluation format.

This chapter presents a format for organizing physical therapy documentation that is based on two important models for physical therapy: the Nagi model of disablement and the patient/client management model from the American Physical Therapy Association's (APTA) *Guide to Physical Therapist Practice*. The format is based on three fundamental assumptions presented in previous chapters: (1) documentation both shapes and reflects clinical problem-solving strategies; (2) a top-down model of disablement provides a useful framework for clinical problem-solving, and thus documentation; and (3) documentation should be organized around functional outcomes.

The format presented herein is intended to provide a set of general guidelines for organizing documentation that can be adapted to different practice settings. It is not intended to be a rigidly applied procedure for writing documentation. PTs practice in a variety of settings, encounter many different types of patients and clients, and write documentation for many different reasons. No single format could be applicable to all these situations. Nevertheless, the general principles of functional outcomes documentation can be captured in a generic format and adapted to different purposes and contexts.

Two main formats for documentation are presented in this book: (1) a format for writing the initial evaluation of a patient and (2) a format for writing progress or daily notes. Other types of documentation, such as discharge summaries, letters to referral sources, and others, can easily be constructed from these two main types. The major focus of this book is on the initial evaluation format because it is the most critical to establishing a framework for clinical problem solving. Each section of the initial evaluation format is further detailed in separate chapters (Chapters 4 to 10). The format for progress and daily notes is a modified form of the *SOAP* note and is presented in Chapter 11. (SOAP is an acronym that stands for the four main sections of this format: *s*ubjective-*o*bjective-*a*ssessment-*p*lan.) Practice exercises in categorizing statements into one of the six sections of the initial evaluation format are provided at the end of this chapter.

The format for an initial evaluation is based on the top-down disablement model presented in Chapter 1. There are six main sections (Table 3-1). The first three sections include information about all four levels of Nagi's disablement model: pathology and disability (Reason for Referral section), functional limitations (Functional Status section), and impairments (Impairment section). The next three sections present the physical therapy diagnosis (Assessment), the Goals, and the Intervention Plan.

One of the important contributions of the APTA's *Guide to Physical Therapist Practice* is the "patient/client management model." This model describes the process by which a PT determines the critical problems that require intervention and develops an intervention plan to address those problems. The model defines five integrated elements of the process: examination, evaluation, diagnosis, prognosis, and intervention. The model is illustrated and each of the elements is defined in Figure 3-1.

The initial evaluation format fits very closely with the patient/client management model (Table 3-2). In this format, examination and evaluation are combined. As is emphasized in the patient/client management model, evaluation is a dynamic process—not something that is initiated only after all data have been collected. Therefore there is an interplay between examination and evaluation. Data are collected and evaluated, and then decisions are made about what additional data to collect. This process often may involve hypothesis testing. In the functional outcomes approach the starting point for data collection is the reason for referral, which establishes both the primary reasons for referral and the patient's disability or potential disability. This then leads to specific examination procedures to determine what functional limitations are producing the disability and what impairments are leading to those functional limitations. Thus the functional outcomes format applies a logical sequence to the reporting of the data that were collected. The data are reported in a framework that reflects a disability-focused (or ability-focused) approach.

The critical step in clinical reasoning is establishing a physical therapy diagnosis. The diagnosis establishes the causes of specific problems that the PT or PTA will address in the intervention strategy. Sometimes the diagnosis may be a statement of the nature and location of the pathologic condition that is causing the problem. More commonly it is a statement of the causal links between impairments and functional limitations. Diagnosis in physical therapy is a relatively new concept and is considered in more detail in Chapter 8.

After a diagnosis has been established, the PT determines the expected outcomes, based on the history, examination, and other factors. In the functional outcomes format these outcomes are organized into three sets of goals: disability goals, functional goals, and impairment goals. This organization clarifies the distinct nature of these goals and encourages the formulation of goals at each level.

In the last section of the initial evaluation the PT plans a strategy for intervention. As noted in the *Guide to Physical Therapist Practice*, intervention involves three processes: coordination and communication, patient-client-related instruction, and procedural interventions. Again, each is given a separate subsection in the initial evaluation format to encourage explicit documentation of these categories.

TABLE 3-1 SIX SECTIONS OF THE INITIAL EVALUATION FORMAT	
Main Section	**Information Included**
Reason for referral	1. Medical diagnosis/history 2. Disability/social history
Functional status	**Performance** in functional **skills** needed to avoid or overcome disability
Impairments	Alterations in **function of body systems** that are linked to observed functional limitations
Assessment	Physical therapy **diagnosis**
Goals	1. **Disability** goals 2. **Functional** goals 3. **Impairment** goals
Intervention plan	1. **Coordination** and **communication** 2. Patient-client related **instruction** 3. Procedural **interventions**

A DESCRIPTION OF THE INITIAL EVALUATION FORMAT

The following sections discuss each of the main components of the initial evaluation format in some detail. Each component is further detailed in Chapters 4 to 10. Case Examples 3-1 and 3-2 (pp. 30-34) provide samples of completed initial evaluations using this format.* Table 3-3 summarizes the evaluation process, emphasizing clinical decision making.

_____

*All cases presented in this book may be loosely based on actual patients. However, all names are fictitious and identifying information has been deleted or changed.

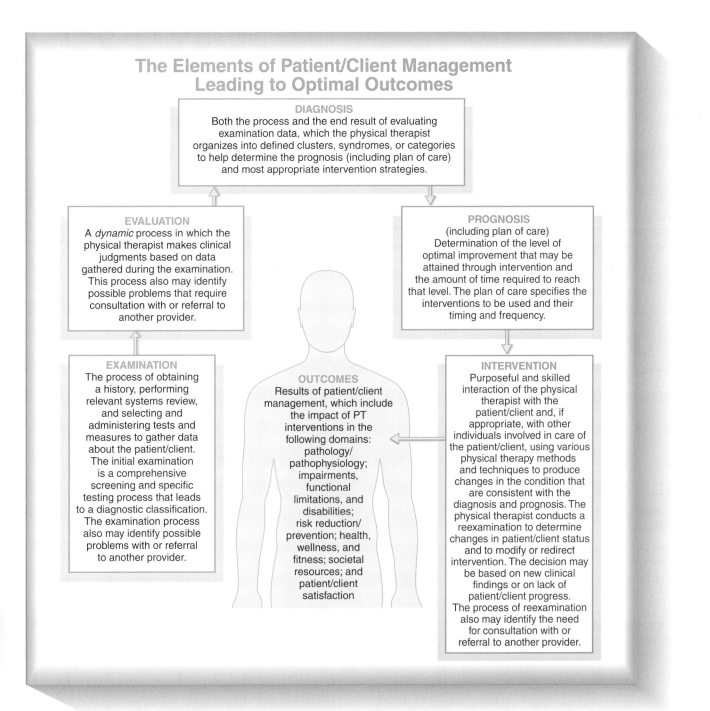

FIGURE 3-1

The patient/client management model.

(Reprinted with permission from the *Guide to Physical Therapist Practice,* 2001.)

TABLE 3-2 FUNCTIONAL OUTCOMES DOCUMENTATION—INITIAL EVALUATION		
Patient/Client Management Model	**Components of the Initial Evaluation**	**Process**
Examination/evaluation	Reason for referral	Explain medical conditions **(pathology)** that are pertinent to patient's disability Determine **disability** or potential disability
	Functional status	Measure patient performance on the **functional** activities that the individual needs to perform to overcome or prevent the disability
	Impairments	Identify and measure the **impairments** that contribute to the observed functional limitations
Diagnosis	Assessment	Establish a physical therapy **diagnosis**—the links between levels of the disablement model, most frequently impairments and functional limitations
Prognosis	Goals	Develop a set of **functional goals** in consultation with the patient
Intervention	Intervention plan	Plan an **intervention strategy** that will help the patient achieve the functional goals

Reason for Referral

Reason for referral typically entails a short narrative summary of the reason for evaluating a particular patient in physical therapy (see Chapters 4 and 5). This includes defining the medical diagnosis and pertinent medical history, as well as the patient's social history and any current disabilities. This information is linked together in this one section as it provides the rationale for why the patient was referred for evaluation. The following two sections are included in Reason for Referral.

Medical Diagnosis and History   The medical diagnosis and history section include the following information (as pertinent, see Chapter 4):

- Patient information, such as name, age, and gender of patient
- Current condition (history of present illness): medical diagnosis/pathology information
- Past medical history, identifying source: patient report, chart review, or both, or other
- Medications

Disability and Social History   The principal purpose of this section is to establish the patient's disability or potential disability, and document pertinent social history (see Chapter 5). *Disability* refers to an inability of an individual to fulfill desired or required personal, social, or occupational roles or to achieve personal goals. *Social history* includes information about a person's living environment and situation (such as where they live and with whom) and their current work or employment situation. This section should also encompass information pertaining to a patient's general health status, including participation, or limitation in participation, in recreational and social activities. It would be pertinent to include information about how the patient's current level of functioning in his or her life roles has changed due to the current medical condition. Standardized outcomes measures of a person's disability are reported in this section. These assess a person's overall quality-of-life or the level of assistance or caregiver burden required to complete life tasks.

Functional Status

Information in the functional status section is intended to identify the critical functional limitations that contribute to the disability (see Chapter 6). What are the

TABLE 3-3 PROCESS USED TO EVALUATE A PATIENT, DETERMINE A DIAGNOSIS, AND DEVELOP A PLAN FOR INTERVENTION

Main Sections of Initial Evaluation	Analysis of Disablement	Conceptualizing Rehabilitation	Questions the Physical Therapist Asks
Reason for referral	Disability	Personal/social roles	• What is the primary medical condition? • How is the current condition affecting the individual's life?
Functional status	Functional limitations	Skill	• What specific functional skills does the individual need to learn (or relearn) in order to be able to accomplish the roles? • How does inadequate performance in specific functional activities prevent the individual from fulfilling life roles? • What specific movement systems are poorly executed (e.g., reach, grasp, gait, balance)?
Impairments	Impairments	Movement/resources	• How are why are the individual's movements dysfunctional? • What neuromuscular or sensorimotor mechanisms are inadequate (e.g., ROM, strength, sensation)?
Assessment	Problem list	Diagnosis	• What are the causal links between functional limitations and disabilities? …between impairments and functional limitations? …between pathology and impairments?
Goals	Prognosis	Objectives of intervention	• What functional goals have the therapist and patient agreed on? • What functional activities will be used to benchmark the patient's progress toward accomplishing the overall goals?
Intervention plan	Treatment	Education	• What musculoskeletal, neuromotor, and physiologic resources must be enhanced to enable the individual to relearn the specified functional skills? • What sequence of tasks will optimally challenge the patient? • What should be done to promote tissue healing or prevent damage?

functional skills that (1) the individual needs to perform to fulfill his or her goals and required roles and (2) are now in some way less than adequate? Functional abilities should be reported concretely and completely, and should be quantified to the degree possible. This can be done by use of quantifiable measurements (such as walking speed or distance walked), or by use of standardized tests that measure functional abilities.

Impairments

This section identifies those impairments, such as range of motion limitations or strength deficits, that have a causal relationship to the observed functional limitations or might cause functional limitations in the future if not treated (see Chapter 7). This information should be documented using objective measures, such as degrees of range of motion or manual muscle testing grade, whenever possible.

Physical Therapy Initial Evaluation
Setting: Outpatient

Name: Smith, Herbert   *D.O.B.:* 6/4/40   *Date of Eval:* 07/29/99

REASON FOR REFERRAL

Current Condition: Mr. Smith is a 59 y.o. male s/p L TKR on 7/21/99. Pt. reports gradually increasing pain in B knees for the last 2-3 yrs, c̄ the L knee becoming severe within the last 2 mos.

Past Medical History: OA B knees diagnosed 3 yrs ago; controlled HTN

Medications: Lopressor, Coumadin, Percocet

Disability/Social History: Pt. lives c̄ wife in 2 story home; 5 steps to enter, 12 steps in between floors (8-inch height). Immediately before surgery pt. was unable to stand s̄ UE support for more than 30 min. Pt. reports walking "very slowly" before surgery and had "sharp" L knee pain when putting weight on L leg. Pt. required arm assistance from wife when walking long distances. At present, pt. in unable to perform household tasks such as cleaning and assisting with house maintenance. Pt.'s wife assists c̄ household tasks and ADLs as needed. Pt. is employed as a surgeon. Before this surgery he worked full time, up to 12 hr days, and was required to stand for up to 1 1/2 hrs at a time. Pt. has not returned to work 2° to standing and walking limitations postsurgery. Pt. reports that for many years he enjoyed playing golf 2×/wk but has been unable to do so for the last 4 mos before surgery 2° to pain and walking limitations.

FUNCTIONAL STATUS

Ambulation: Walks c̄ 2 straight canes using 4-point gait pattern c̄ supervision for indoor distances; can walk 50 ft in 60 sec before needing to sit 2° to pain. Pt. demonstrates ↓ L stance time and antalgic gait pattern. Has not attempted outdoor ambulation.

Stair Climbing: ↑↓ 12 steps of 8-inch height using arm railing and 1 str cane c̄ step-to-step pattern c̄ supervision within 2 min; unable to negotiate stairs using a step-over-step pattern.

Self-Care: Pt reports he is I in dressing x̄ requires min A to don/doff L sock and shoe. Pt. reports he showers in a stall shower holding onto grab bar; needs min A of wife (to reach LEs and occasionally to maintain balance).

Standing Tasks: Able to stand for 10 min at countertop (kitchen or bathroom) while reaching c̄ either hand, using other hand for support. No limitations in reaching for objects above shoulder height. Unable to reach for objects below knee height to either side.

IMPAIRMENTS

ROM
AROM knee ext L –18°, R –10°; flex L 18-68°, R 10-100°; ankle DF L –5°, R 0-5°
PROM knee ext L –13°, R –5°; flex L 13-75°, R 5-105°; ankle DF L 0°, R 0-10°

Strength
L knee ext: 4/5; R knee ext: 5/5
L knee flex: 4/5; R knee flex: 4+/5

Anthropometric Measurements: Height 5' 8"; weight 220 lbs; circumferential measurements: mid-patella L > R by 1.5", mid-malleoli L > R by 0.75"

Pain: Pt. has experienced pain around entire L knee joint since surgery 8 days ago; gradually improving. Pain at rest is described as "aching" (3/10 on VAS), c̄ occasional "sharp" pain c̄ weight bearing (6/10 on VAS), and at end range of motion (8/10). Pain in R knee 2/10 described as "constant, dull pain."

Integumentary: Observation reveals L knee is edematous c̄ significant rubor, surgical site is clean, dry, and intact c̄ steri-strips in place. No observable exudates present.

Systems Review
- Resting vitals: HR 76 bpm; BP 128/84 mm Hg; RR 16
- Vitals post ambulation (50 ft): HR 84 bpm; BP 132/84 mm Hg; RR 22
- (+) blood supply and venous return in distal L LE
- No evidence of cognitive or neurologic impairments; able to communicate effectively

Continued

CASE EXAMPLE 3-1

Physical Therapy Initial Evaluation—cont'd
Setting: Outpatient

Name: Smith, Herbert   *D.O.B.:* 6/4/40   *Date of Eval:* 07/29/99

ASSESSMENT

Pt. is a 59 y.o. male, moderately obese, s/p L TKR who presents c̄ limitations in L knee ROM and strength and postsurgical edema. This has resulted in an inability to ambulate and climb stairs independently, c̄ reduced speed and limited distance, and limited independence in dressing and bathing. Edema, pain, and ↓ L knee strength have also resulted in reduced ability to bear weight on his L side, which is evident by pt.'s impaired gait pattern and standing tolerance. Pain and ↓ R knee strength 2° to OA may additionally limit pt.'s functional recovery. Pt. requires outpatient PT to address these impairments and functional limitations to facilitate functional independence and return to work and previous recreational activities.

GOALS

Disability Goals
1. Pt. will return to work at the same capacity as 6 months ago, within 4 mos.
2. Pt. will be able to play golf twice/wk, walk 9 holes, ride for 9 holes, within 4 mos.

Functional Goals
1. Pt. will be able to don/doff shoes and socks independently 3/3 days within 1 wk.
2. Pt. will ambulate 500 ft inside clinic corridors, gait speed at least 1.0 m/sec without an assistive device independently within 2 wks.
3. Pt. will ↑ 4 flights of stairs (48 stairs; 8″ height) using a railing and step-over-step pattern in less than 5 minutes, within 3 wks.
4. Pt. will ambulate outside over curbs and on grass independently using a str cane within 4 wks.
5. Pt. will stand for 30 min while performing UE activities at a countertop within 4 wks.

Impairment Goals
1. Pain will be less than 3/10 in L knee during weight-bearing activities within 2 wks.
2. AROM L knee ext will increase to –5°, L knee flex to 5-90° within 3 wks.
3. PROM L knee ext will increase to 0°, L knee flex to 0-100° within 3 wks.
4. Strength B knee flex will increase to 5/5 within 3 wks.
5. Strength L knee ext will increase to 5/5 within 3 wks.

INTERVENTION PLAN

Pt. will be seen 3 ×/wk for 45 min each session. Pt. will be re-evaluated in 4 wks.

Coordination/Communication
Order will be placed through medical supplier for shower chair for stall shower.

Patient-Related Instruction
Pt. instructed in pain/edema management activities c̄ elevation and ice, therapeutic exercises emphasizing quadriceps and hamstring flexibility, strength and function in both open and closed kinetic chains (supine, seated and standing). Patient also instructed in safety precautions on stairs and uneven surfaces. Patient verbalized understanding of all instructions. Will continue to progress pt. c̄ HEP, and instruct pt. in importance of proper diet and long-term exercise.

Procedural Interventions
Cryotherapy to L knee followed by quadriceps/hamstring/calf stretching and A/PROM activities in supine, sitting and standing to B knees. Gait trng indoors and outdoors on a variety of surfaces and inclines to improve safety, endurance, speed, and ↓ need for assistive device. Stair climbing trng to improve endurance and independence. Practice of a variety of activities incorporating UEs in standing (including kitchen tasks, self-care activities, and golf swings) to improve standing tolerance, knee strength, and stability.

The findings of this evaluation were discussed c̄ the patient, and he consented to the above intervention plan.

_____   _____
Jen L. Therapist   Date

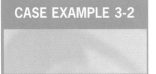

Physical Therapy Initial Evaluation

Setting: Inpatient Rehabilitation

Name: Rizzo, Rachel   *D.O.B.:* 2/7/53   *Date of Eval:* 07/10/99

REASON FOR REFERRAL

Current Condition: Pt. is a 46 y.o. female admitted to County Rehabilitation Center on 7/9/99 c̄ diagnosis of exacerbation of multiple sclerosis (initial diagnosis 1996). Pt. admitted to County acute care hospital 7/4/99 for IV steroid treatment. Referral by primary MD requests gait training 2° to recent exacerbation leading to difficulty walking.

Past Medical History: R ACL repair 15 yrs ago.

Medications: Prednisone, Avonex, Baclofen

Disability/Social History: Currently, pt. needs A for general mobility and some ADLs. Before this hospitalization, she performed ADLs independently and ambulated with a str cane. Pt. lived c̄ her 21 y.o. son in a ground floor apartment c̄ no steps. She was responsible for light housekeeping and some cooking. Her son assisted c̄ some housekeeping and daily chores, and states he is available to assist c̄ other tasks as needed when she returns home. Pt. has not been employed for past year 2° to disability; pt. reports fatigue is 1° limiting factor. Pt. volunteers 1 day/wk for 4 hrs at local library sorting books and assisting c̄ computer searches.

FUNCTIONAL STATUS

Bed Mobility: Pt. positions self comfortably in bed and rolls B l'ly. Supine ↔ sitting on bed c̄ min A for LEs.

Transfers: Pt. transfers from sit → stand from bed c̄ min A. She uses both arms to assist c̄ push off but needs A to get to standing. Transfers from w/c ↔ bed c̄ min A using rolling walker; able to transfer c̄ CG c̄ use of SB l'ly.

Sitting Ability: Sitting balance on edge of bed can be maintained erect for 5 min s̄ UE support (limited due to self-reported fatigue). Can sit l'ly in W/C for > 30 min.

Standing Ability: Pt. stands for up to 3 min. c̄ rolling walker. Can stand at bathroom sink and perform simple one-handed self-care activities. Uses R arm to maintain balance.

Mobility: Pt. walks 50 feet c̄ rolling walker and min A on a smooth floor hospital corridor in 2:25 min (average 2 trials). HR increased to 130 bpm. Pt. can propel wheelchair for distances in hospital corridor up to 100 ft, after which she reports fatigue.

Bathing: Requires mod A from nurse's aide to transfer in and out of tub, and to bathe completely. Needs to sit down while bathing 2° to fatigue.

IMPAIRMENTS

Muscle Tone: Modified Ashworth Scale 2/4 B hip adductors and gastrocs.

Sensation: Impaired sensation to light touch (5/8 correct responses) and pin prick (4/8 correct responses) below knees B.

Strength

	Left	Right
Hip flexion	2/5	3/5
Hip extension	2/5	3/5
Hip abduction	2+/5	3/5
Hip adduction	3/5	3/5
Knee extension	3–/5	3+/5
Knee flexion	3/5	3/5
Ankle dorsiflexion	2/5	3/5
Ankle plantarflexion	2/5	3/5

PROM
- Hip abd: L 0-25°; R 0-30°
- Ankle DF L 0°; R 0-5°

Gait Impairments: Pt. has difficulty advancing her L leg during swing; requires min A 25% of the time. Stride length is decreased B, ↓ stance time and WB on L LE. Pt. exhibits Trendelenburg gait to compensate for L abd. weakness during L stance.

Continued

CASE EXAMPLE 3-2

Physical Therapy Initial Evaluation—cont'd
Setting: Inpatient Rehabilitation

Name: Rizzo, Rachel   *D.O.B.:* 2/7/53   *Date of Eval:* 07/10/99

Balance: Berg Balance Score: 7/56

Sitting: Pt. can reach 5 inches outside arm's length to the front and to both sides. Pt. able to maintain balance to mod. external perturbations c̄ independent recovery in all directions (5/5 trials).

Standing: Pt. can reach only 3 inches outside arm's length to the front and both sides. Pt. able to maintain balance to mod anterior and posterior perturbations 3/5 trials; stepping strategy used 2/3 trials to posterior perturbation. Pt. is able to stand for 10 sec s̄ walker; reports that she is fearful of falling.

Fatigue: Pt. reports fatigue as avg. 6.5/7 on Fatigue Severity Scale (scale 1-7, 7 = highest severity). Pt. feels fatigue has worsened since recent exacerbation.

Skin Assessment: Edema noted in B ankles, L < R (28 cm circumference L malleoli, 26 cm on R).

Pain: No reports of pain

Systems Review: HR 72 bpm; BP 130/84 mm Hg, RR 20 at rest. Pt. reports STM loss, mild deficit noted during interview and evaluation. Able to communicate effectively.

ASSESSMENT

Pt. is a 46 y.o. female who presents c̄ exacerbation of MS symptoms. Pt presents c̄ LE weakness, impaired balance, fatigue, and limited PROM B hip abd and ankle DF, which have led to limitations in performing bed mobility, self-care, and ambulation. Limited endurance and LE weakness have led to limitations in pt. using ambulation as her primary means of mobility. Pt. requires inpatient rehabilitation to address this recent decline in functional abilities and to assist patient in returning to prior functional level.

GOALS

Disability Goal
1. Pt. will carry out self-care activities and mobility within the home c̄ no greater than min A of a home health aide in her apartment within 1 month.

Functional Goals
1. Pt. will rise from supine → sitting position on edge of bed I'ly 5/5 trials within 20 sec (1 wk).
2. Pt. will maintain sitting position on edge of bed for 10 min I'ly (1 wk).
3. Pt. will transfer from sitting on bed → standing (c̄ walker) I'ly, 5/5 trials (1 wk).
4. Pt. will stand for 10 min at bathroom sink while performing self care tasks (2 wks).
5. Pt. will walk 200 ft within 2 min, in hospital hallway c̄ supervision using a rollator, c̄ HR < 110 bpm (2 wks).

INTERVENTION PLAN

Pt. will be seen b.i.d. 7 days/wk during rehab stay. Full reeval in 2 wks. PT should continue on q.d. basis s/p DC.

Coordination/Communication
Practice in bathing and other self-care activities will be coordinated c̄ the OT Department. Will request order of compression stockings from physician and training in proper use via Nursing. Consider referral to orthotic clinic within 1-2 wks for possible L AFO.

Patient-Related Instruction
Pt. and nursing aides will be instructed in optimal strategies for performing functional activities, esp. transfers. Pt. and family will be instructed in evening and weekend exercise routine to increase PROM hip abd. & ankle DF, and receive instruction for guarding during transfers and ambulation. Fatigue management and energy conservation discussed c̄ pt., and will continue to be incorporated t/o PT sessions.

Direct Interventions
Stretching exercises to ↑ PROM hip abd and ankle DF. AROM and strengthening exercises in supine and standing for B LE musculature, focusing on hip √ and abd, knee, and ankle PF/DF. Trng in bed mobility, transfers and sitting ability (to increase endurance). Standing balance trng to address standing balance limitations, and improve endurance. Gait trng in different environments to improve speed, safety and endurance, and decrease need for physical assistance. Progress pt. with assistive device to use of a 4-wheeled rollator, to consider for home use.

The findings of this evaluation were discussed c̄ the patient, and she consented to the above intervention plan.

_____   _____
Jen L. Therapist   Date

Assessment

The assessment section typically begins with an overall impression: a brief statement summarizing the patient's reason for being referred for physical therapy. Next, the PT puts forth a PT diagnosis, which is the major component of the assessment. The PT diagnosis entails the reason or reasons why certain functional limitations are present (see Chapter 9). Normally this diagnosis will link either a pathologic condition or impairment to functional limitations. APTA *Guidelines for Physical Therapy Documentation* state that a physical therapy diagnosis is required for all initial evaluations. The assessment concludes with a statement summarizing the PT's general recommendations.

Problem List (Optional)   Often a list of a set of "problems" that link specific impairments to functional limitations is useful. Such a problem list is indicated when the patient has several distinct functional problems, each caused by different impairments. Each problem is really a separate diagnosis.

If a problem list is used, it should be prioritized (i.e., first problem on the list is most important or the first one to be addressed).

Goals

This section identifies the expected outcomes of physical therapy intervention, the ends toward which physical therapy intervention is directed (see Chapter 9). Specific *goals* are written that are related to these outcomes. The goals can have several levels:

Disability Goals Typically one or two disability goals are useful to highlight the overall level of function patient is expected to achieve. Disability goals need not be measurable in a strict sense.

Functional Goals Functional goals state the predicted functional performance at the end of therapy. These goals must be measurable and include specific time frames.

Impairment Goals (Therapy Goals) Impairment goals document expected improvements or changes in impairments that will result at the end of therapy. These goals should have a clear relationship to the stated functional goals. For example, achieving a certain shoulder range of motion may be critical to the functional task of lifting or reaching. This relationship need not be documented in detail with each impairment goal but should be documented as part of the Assessment.

DOCUMENTATION OF GOALS

All three levels of goals are *not* required for each documentation. The type and number of goals written depends on the setting and context. However, at a minimum, functional goals should be included in an initial evaluation documentation.

Intervention Plan

This section outlines the plan for achieving the goals listed in the previous section and presents a concise rationale for the intervention strategy chosen. It is useful to begin with the proposed frequency of treatments, as well as a tentative date for reevaluation. Many institutions mandate this approach. The intervention plan should then be documented in the following three categories.

Coordination and Communication   Services that require coordination or communication with other providers, agencies, departments, and so on should be included here.

Patient- or Client-Related Instruction   The PT should document specific instruction or teaching of the patient or of the patient's caregivers.

Procedural Interventions
These interventions are direct interventions performed by the PT or PTA (e.g., therapeutic exercise, functional training, and manual therapy techniques). (See Figure 10-1 for appropriate categorization and terminology from the *Guide*.)

CONCLUSION

This chapter has outlined the initial evaluation format for functional outcomes documentation. This format is designed so that physical therapy documentation reflects the evaluative, diagnostic, and planning processes that PTs and PTAs use in modern practice. Indeed, as evident in the Guide to Physical Therapist Practice, practice is moving from a format based on medical models to a more patient-centered, disability-oriented approach. The format outlined in this chapter attempts to capture both of these aspects of physical therapy practice (see Table 3-3).

Two examples are included to illustrate how the initial evaluation format might be used in actual practice (see Case Examples 3-1 and 3-2). Readers, especially beginning students, should not see this format as a rigid blueprint to be copied exactly in other situations. Rather, this format should be perceived as a starting point, a set of guidelines to be used for designing effective physical therapy documentation.

SUMMARY

■ The format for writing functional outcomes reports is based on (1) clinical problem-solving strategies, (2) a top-down model of disablement, and (3) organization around functional outcomes.

■ The format provides a set of general guidelines that can be adapted to different practice settings.

■ The format has six main sections: reason for referral, functional status, impairments, assessment, goals, and intervention plan (see Table 3-1).

■ The critical step in the evaluation process and clinical reasoning is establishing a physical therapy diagnosis. The diagnosis states the causal links between impairments and functional limitations and disability. The diagnosis therefore establishes the specific problems that the PT or PTA will address in the intervention strategy.

EXERCISE 3-1

In the space provided, identify in which of the six sections of the initial evaluation model each of the following statements belong (R = Reason for Referral; F = Functional Status; I = Impairments; A = Assessment; G = Goals; IP = Intervention Plan). The statements are taken from a variety of initial evaluation reports.

1. Child will ride an adaptive tricycle independently for 25 feet in the gym in 8 weeks. _G_

2. ROM R knee flexion 95°. _I_

3. BP 150/90, HR 96. _I_

4. Pt. has a 2-yr history of seizures occurring approximately 2 ×/month. _R_

5. Pt. education will include instructions in home program for walking program with self-monitoring of HR and perceived exertion. _IP_

6. Pt. works as a secretary full time but is only able to work part-time (1/2 days) due to wrist pain. _R_

7. Pt. is able to climb 10 stairs with left hand holding railing in 25 seconds. _F_

8. Pt. presents with poor expiratory ability 2° to pneumonia, resulting in an ineffective cough and lowered endurance for daily care activities. _A_

9. Pt. is a 23-year-old professional dancer who works 7 days/week. _R_

10. Pt. will be able to stand at bathroom sink for 5 minutes to brush teeth and wash face and comb hair in 2 weeks. _G_

11. Intervention will include therapeutic exercise: progressive resistive exercises to quadriceps and strengthening in standing position via squatting and lunging exercises. _IP_

12. Strength R shoulder flexion 3+/5. _I_

13. The pt's. ineffective right toe clearance and weak hip musculature are resulting in slow and unsafe ambulation indoors. _F_

14. Pt. can lift a 10-lb. box (maximum weight) from floor to waist height. _F_

15. Therapist will coordinate training for dressing and bathing with patient's OT and with nursing staff. _IP_

Components of Physical Therapy Documentation

CHAPTER 4

Documenting Reason for Referral: Background Information, Medical Diagnosis, and History

LEARNING OBJECTIVES

After reading this chapter and completing the exercises, the reader will be able to:

1. Identify three sources where medical diagnosis and pathology information pertaining to a patient can be obtained.

2. Identify and classify various aspects of documenting a patient's background information, medical diagnosis, and past medical history.

3. Appropriately document components of a patient's background information, medical diagnosis, and past medical history.

4. Describe the three key elements of describing a pathologic or medical condition.

5. Discuss the implications of direct access for documenting medical diagnoses.

Within the scope of their practice, physical therapists encounter patients with a variety of pathologic conditions. Pathology can result from conditions such as infection, acute injury, metabolic imbalance, or degenerative disease processes. Nagi (1991) refers to pathology as "diagnoses of disease, injury, congenital/developmental condition." Any physical therapy initial evaluation note must provide specific information about the medical diagnosis or known or suspected pathologic conditions. Because they may be pertinent to the patient's referral to physical therapy, the pathologic condition and medical diagnosis must be presented in a clear and concise fashion in the PT's documentation.

In the *Guide to Physical Therapist Practice*, pathologic information is categorized under "History" in the Examination Section. The *Guide* defines history as follows:

The history is a systematic gathering of data—from both the past and the present—related to why the patient/client is seeking the services of the physical therapist....While taking the history, the physical

therapist also identifies health restoration and prevention needs and coexisting health problems that may have implications for intervention (*Guide to Physical Therapist Practice*, 2001, p. S34).

Thus the relevance of history taking, as it relates to pathologic conditions and medical diagnoses, is that it provides the foundation for the reason for referral. What are the specific medical diagnoses, underlying pathologic conditions, health problems, or health risk factors that bring the patient to seek the services of a physical therapist?

This chapter expands on the concept of the reason for referral as it relates to pathologic conditions and medical diagnosis. Students will have an opportunity to practice writing statements related to medical diagnosis and history and appropriately identify information that belongs in this section of a report. Chapter 5 discusses how information obtained about a person's disability and social history further contributes to determining reason for referral.

DOCUMENTING ELEMENTS OF PATHOLOGIC CONDITIONS

In general, pathology information and the medical diagnosis are included early in an evaluation because these data are critical to determining how the PT should proceed with the examination. Certain conditions raise concerns about whether an underlying condition exists in which physical therapy may be contraindicated and in which referral to another health professional would be warranted.

Pathology information is therefore an important part of determining the *appropriateness* of physical therapy as an intervention. Certain medical conditions are appropriate for physical therapy; others are not. However, medical diagnosis alone does not determine the appropriateness of intervention; instead, it is the associated or secondary limitations or impairments related to a medical diagnosis that warrant physical therapy intervention. It should be noted, however, that the PT does not simply accept the medical diagnosis as the whole story. An important part of the PT's role in determining the appropriateness of physical therapy is to perform a systems review. Therapists will ask pathology-related questions, which help to identify possible problems that require consultation with or referral to another provider.

Thus the pathology information documented by the PT in this section is limited. At this point the therapist simply classifies any facts he or she has available before the examination is performed. As the examination proceeds, the PT may uncover information that may help to refine the diagnosis. Any new information obtained during the course of the physical therapy examination that confirms, clarifies, elaborates on, or possibly contradicts the established medical diagnosis and pathology information should be documented in the appropriate section (e.g., Impairments) and summarized in the Assessment section (see Chapter 8). Thus information about pathologic conditions and medical diagnosis does not begin and end in this section.

Pathology information can be organized in the initial evaluation note in many ways. Different institutions frequently mandate a certain organizational structure, and this is often preprinted on customized initial evaluation forms. For the general initial evaluation, the following categorization of information is recommended to document pathology and the reason for referral:

- Patient information
- Current condition
- Past medical history
- Medications
- Other (family or developmental history, as pertinent)

The degree to which each of these headings is used may differ depending on the institution and patient population. Next, documentation of information in each of these categories is discussed. Figure 4-1 provides a detailed listing of the types of information that can be included in each of these categories. Case Examples 4-1, 4-2, and 4-3 provide sample documentation in different clinical settings.

Types of Information to Be Documented

Patient Information and Demographics General patient information and demographics are the first items included in any medical documentation and typically include the patient's name, age, date of birth, and any pertinent demographic information. If the patient's race or ethnic background is relevant to the patient's diagnosis, it can be included here. This section also may include information pertaining to why the patient or client was referred for physical therapy and by whom if it is not evident. This sets the framework for the reason this evaluation is being performed.

Current Condition This section of the report should include information about the *current medical condition* (medical diagnosis) for which the patient is being referred for physical therapy. In fact, this section of a note is often simply titled "medical diagnosis." In most cases the PT should go beyond simply restating the medical diagnosis and describe a specific precipitating incident, if any, or mechanism of injury (MOI). The therapist should also report what other treatments have been performed (e.g., consultation with other medical professionals). If the specific medical condition is not known, the therapist should document any information provided by the patient identifying the primary problem or *chief complaint—* what is the reason the patient is seeking the PT's services?

Whenever possible, documentation should include *specific* pathology information that is helpful in understanding the nature of the problem and making a physical therapy diagnosis. In many situations in physical therapy, information about the patient's pathologic condition is obtained through the medical diagnosis, which often is provided by the referring physician. Many exceptions exist, particularly for admittedly frequent cases in which the medical diagnosis is simply a statement of the patient's problem (e.g., "low back pain").

Information about the patient's pathologic condition sets the foundation for the physical therapy examination. The PT must gather all relevant information to develop an accurate picture of the patient's medical condition that warrants referral to physical therapy. Whenever possible, three key elements of pathology/ medical condition should be specified: underlying disease process, location, and time course (Figure 4-2).

COMPONENTS OF DOCUMENTING REASON FOR REFERRAL: BACKGROUND INFORMATION, MEDICAL DIAGNOSIS & HISTORY

Patient information and demographics

- Patient's name
- Age/date of birth
- Sex
- Demographic information, such as race or ethnicity if relevant
- Reason patient is referred, if not evident

Currrent condition

- Concerns that led the patient to seek the services of a physical therapist
- Concerns or needs of patient who requires the services of a physical therapist
- Current therapeutic interventions
- Mechanisms of injury or disease, including:
  - Underlying disease process
  - Time course
  - Location
- Onset and pattern of symptoms
- Previous occurrence of current condition
- Prior therapeutic interventions

Past medical history

- Prior hospitalizations, surgeries and pre-existing medical and other health-related conditions

Medications

- Medications for current condition
- Medications previously taken for current condition
- Medications for other conditions
- Over-the-counter medication

Other (if applicable)

- Growth and development
  - Developmental history
  - Hand dominance
- Family history
  - Familial health risks

FIGURE 4-1

Components of documenting reason for referral: patient information, current condition, past medical history, medications and other. This figure attempts to incorporate terminology found in the *Guide to Physical Therapist Practice*, 2001, p. S36.

CASE EXAMPLE 4-1	**Documenting Reason for Referral: Background Information, Medical Diagnosis, and History**

Setting: Outpatient

Name: Ally McCarthy   *D.O.B.:* 9/25/35   *Date:* 12/11/00

Patient information: Ally McCarthy is a 65 y.o. female who was referred for PT by Dr. Hull, orthopedic surgeon, for evaluation and intervention related to low back dysfunction.

Current condition: Pt. reports sudden onset of low back pain after lifting heavy boxes 10 days ago. Pt. sought medical advice from Dr. Hull 3 days later on 12/4/00. Dr. Hull prescribed x-rays, which revealed L2-5 DDD as per phone conversation with Dr. Hull. Pt. was then prescribed Flexoril and referred to PT.

Past medical history: Pt. reports the following: NIDDM × 5 yrs; R ACL reconstruction Nov. 1990; no complications and no limitations on activities related to this surgery.

Medications: Flexoril

ELEMENTS OF MEDICAL DIAGNOSIS

Underlying disease process - Identify the type of pathology, such as infection, tumor, trauma, etc. Include the results of any diagnostic tests (such as lab tests, MRI or X-rays), and any information provided directly from the referring physician that identifies the specific pathology.

Location - Specify where the pathology is originating. This might include the specific area of the brain, spinal cord, muscles, nerves, joints or tissues that are affected.

Time course - Specify how long the problem has existed, including date of injury or surgery, or the date a medical diagnosis was made.

FIGURE 4-2

Elements of medical diagnosis.

If a physician or other health care professional referred the patient to physical therapy, this information should be documented in this section. If applicable, the name of the referring professional should also be listed here in addition to any specific information, orders, or contraindications that he or she communicated.

Past Medical History Information documented in this category should include any medical history that may be relevant (even indirectly) to the current condition. This could include any prior surgeries, other medical diagnoses, or preexisting conditions (such as insulin-dependent diabetes mellitus [IDDM] or history of heart disease). Indicating a date of a surgery (e.g., ACL repair May 1999) or time frame of a medical condition (e.g., IDDM × 10 yrs.) is useful.

Medications Therapists should document medications the patient is taking for the current condition, as well as any medications taken for other medical conditions. Vitamins and over-the-counter medica-tions may also be included, especially if they have known side effects that would be important to consider.

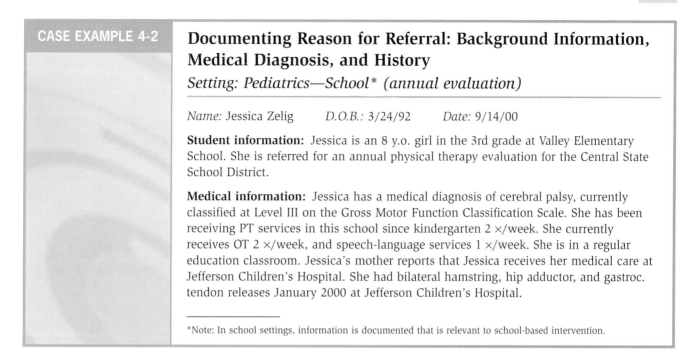

CASE EXAMPLE 4-2

Documenting Reason for Referral: Background Information, Medical Diagnosis, and History

Setting: Pediatrics—School* (annual evaluation)

Name: Jessica Zelig   *D.O.B.:* 3/24/92   *Date:* 9/14/00

Student information: Jessica is an 8 y.o. girl in the 3rd grade at Valley Elementary School. She is referred for an annual physical therapy evaluation for the Central State School District.

Medical information: Jessica has a medical diagnosis of cerebral palsy, currently classified at Level III on the Gross Motor Function Classification Scale. She has been receiving PT services in this school since kindergarten 2 ×/week. She currently receives OT 2 ×/week, and speech-language services 1 ×/week. She is in a regular education classroom. Jessica's mother reports that Jessica receives her medical care at Jefferson Children's Hospital. She had bilateral hamstring, hip adductor, and gastroc. tendon releases January 2000 at Jefferson Children's Hospital.

*Note: In school settings, information is documented that is relevant to school-based intervention.

Other Information Several other types of information most appropriately belong in this section of a report. These include developmental history and family history. A developmental history can be used in certain pediatric settings and involves information related to a child's growth and overall development (e.g., the age at which a child first sat up or walked alone). This information would not be pertinent, however, for most adolescent or adult evaluations. A family history may be helpful for understanding the patient's medical diagnosis (e.g., a strong family history of heart disease or a history of certain musculoskeletal abnormalities).

OBTAINING MEDICAL DIAGNOSIS INFORMATION

Information about the patient's medical diagnosis and history can be obtained in different ways. First, the information can be obtained directly from the physician, either by referring to the medical record or by personal communication. Second, it can be provided directly by the patient, but this method can be less reliable than obtaining it directly from medical personnel or a medical record. Third, information can be obtained through a third party such as a family member. This method is useful when the patient is unable to provide an accurate account of his or her own medical condition.

Because of the differences in how pathology information and medical history can be obtained, documentation of the source(s) of information is important and should be made in this section. For example, if infor-

mation about a patient's medical history is obtained directly from the patient, the PT could write "Pt. reports having had a L ACL reconstruction in 1996." Otherwise, those who read the record typically assume that the information is obtained from medical personnel or a medical record. Ideally an evaluation report should include information obtained from both the patient (or caregiver/family member) and medical record or personnel to provide the most comprehensive and complete accounting of the patient's current medical status.

Medical Diagnoses and Direct Access

Therapists who practice in direct-access states face additional issues regarding medical diagnoses. In certain situations under direct access, no medical diagnosis is available. Therapists must then determine the diagnosis and possible pathologic condition through their own evaluation. In some cases this is not possible within the scope of tests and measures available to PTs, and referral to a physician or other health care personnel is warranted. Reports from diagnostic tests such as magnetic resonance imaging scans (MRIs) and x-ray films may be necessary to clarify the patient's pathologic condition.

All PTs, but particularly those who practice in direct-access states, must clearly document all known aspects of a patient's pathologic status and must be able to make a reasonable differential diagnosis. An important question that each therapist must ask is "Is the pathology one that is within the scope of practice for a physical therapist, and is it amenable to physical therapy intervention?" Therefore clear, concise, and accurate documentation of the pathologic status (including disease process, location, and time course) is of utmost importance. In direct-access cases in which the patient has not been referred by a physician, aspects of the medical condition obtained from a patient/family interview and chart review should be documented in this first section of the note. However, the PT's final diagnosis should not be documented until the Assessment section, because it may depend on physical findings not yet presented.

PREVENTION AND HEALTH PROMOTION

Many therapists are currently involved with prevention: primary, secondary, and tertiary. This raises specific issues regarding documentation. For primary prevention, there is not a presenting medical diagnosis or illness. For example, if a therapist performs an evaluation or intervention for a client who is at risk for developing osteoporosis, documentation of pathology information should include *why* the client is at risk for developing this problem and a discussion of the potential consequences.

Secondary and tertiary prevention are related to current disease processes. Secondary prevention consists of decreasing the duration of illness, severity of disease, and sequelae through early diagnosis (see Figure 1-5). This would apply, for example, to individuals with certain types of cardiac disease. Tertiary prevention consists of limiting the degree of disability and promoting rehabilitation and restoration of function in patients with chronic and irreversible diseases, such as multiple sclerosis. Documentation in such cases needs to focus on not just the specific referring pathologic condition (e.g., multiple sclerosis), but on subsequent pathologic conditions and/or impairments that can be prevented (e.g., muscle contractures). This can be a tricky situation because documentation of prevention is not always well accepted by insurance companies. However, the more that therapists can document the need for and purpose of preventative intervention, the more likely it will become standard practice.

SUMMARY

- Medical information, including current condition and past medical history, provides the foundation for the reason for referral.

- Medical information and the medical diagnosis are included early in an evaluation report because of their importance in shaping the therapist's examination.

- Information in this section of the PT's report can typically be organized into the following categories: patient information and demographics, current condition, past medical history, and medications.

- Documentation of *specific* pathology information is important; this includes providing information about the underlying disease process, the location of the pathologic condition, and its time course.

| CASE EXAMPLE 4-3 | **Documenting Reason for Referral: Background Information, Medical Diagnosis, and History** |

Setting: Acute rehabilitation

Name: Tara Smith   *D.O.B.:* 6/19/70   *Date:* 10/4/00

Patient information: Tara Smith is a 30 y.o. female who was admitted to North Haven Rehabilitation Center on 10/3/00 for multidisciplinary rehab.

Current condition: Pt. sustained an incomplete ASIA D C6 SCI s/p MVA 9/24/00. She was sent to North Haven Hospital and stayed there for 9 days. X-rays and MRI revealed a nondisplaced fx of C6 vertebral body requiring no surgical intervention. Referral received for Philadelphia cervical collar when OOB with no active or passive ROM to C-spine and no heavy lifting (> 5 lb).

Past Medical History: Pt. denies any significant PMH; confirmed by chart review.

Medications: Colace and Tylenol

EXERCISE 4-1

Identify the errors in the following statements documenting Reason for Referral (patient information, current condition, past medical history, and medications). Errors could include disease process, location, or time course not specified; not enough detail; or negative connotation or labeling. Indicate the specific word or words that are problematic, if applicable. Rewrite a more appropriate statement in the space provided.

Statement	What Is Wrong?	Rewrite Statement
EXAMPLE: Patient has a strained muscle.	Location of muscle not identified; more detail regarding nature of strain could be provided, if known	Pt. has grade II strain of R quadriceps, sustained 10/1/00
1. Pt. had surgery yesterday.		
2. Pt. reports pain.		
3. Pt. is a young male amputee.		
4. Pt. had a right-sided stroke.		
5. Kelly's mother reports that there is family history of hip problems.		
6. Pt. is taking multiple medications for various medical conditions.		
7. Pt. has amyotrophic lateral sclerosis.		
8. Pt. has typical problems related to aging.		
9. Pt. is taking anti-spasticity meds.		

Continued

Statement	What Is Wrong?	Rewrite Statement
10. Pt. has a family hx of heart problems.		
11. Pt. complains of fatigue.		
12. Referring physician reports that pt. may need to have surgery.		
13. Pt. has a broken leg.		
14. Pt. has cancer.		
15. Jenny's mother reports that she began crawling and walking late.		

EXERCISE 4-2

The following statements are taken from various sections of an initial evaluation report at a pediatric rehabilitation center. Extract the information that would be appropriate to include in this section of the report (Reason for Referral: patient information, current condition, past medical history, medications or other). Indicate those statements that do not belong in this section. Rewrite this information under the appropriate subheadings in the space provided at the end. The sentences should flow together smoothly.

1. Chelsea's mother, Mrs. Green, provided background information regarding Chelsea's past medical history.

2. Chelsea has significant weakness in her arms and legs.

3. Chelsea first began showing symptoms of myotonic dystrophy when she was in 3rd grade.

4. She is not currently taking any medications.

5. Chelsea enjoys math and art classes at school.

6. There is a history of myotonic dystrophy in Chelsea's family, so Mrs. Green and Chelsea were very familiar with related symptoms and problems.

7. Chelsea was referred by the Smithtown School District for this independent PT evaluation to assist in educational planning.

8. Chelsea has not had any surgeries and has not been hospitalized for any reason.

9. Chelsea is able to ascend and descend a full flight of stairs.

10. Chelsea is a 12 y.o. girl who attends Jonesbridge Middle School.

11. Chelsea has a diagnosis of myotonic dystrophy, a form of muscular dystrophy resulting in muscle weakness and accompanied by myotonia (delayed relaxation of muscles after contraction).

12. Chelsea's primary concern is that she gets fatigued when walking between classes.

Background information: _____

_____

_____

_____

Current condition: _____

_____

_____

_____

Past medical history: _____

_____

Medications: _____

_____

Other: _____

_____

Statements that do not belong in this section (statement numbers): _____

_____

CHAPTER 5

Documenting Reason for Referral: Disability and Social History

LEARNING OBJECTIVES

After reading this chapter and completing the exercises, the reader will be able to:

1. Describe the three categories of disability documentation and cite examples of the type of information that should be included under each.
2. Describe the two primary ways that disability can be measured and documented.
3. Identify and classify various aspects of documenting patient disability and social history.
4. Describe the three ways that disability and social history information can be obtained.
5. Appropriately document components of disability and social history.

Documentation at the *disability level* addresses the ability of a patient or client to perform the specific functions pertinent to their everyday life. How is the current condition affecting the individual's life? Is the patient able to perform his or her roles as a husband/wife or father/mother? Is he or she an independently functioning member of society? Can he or she work, in either a paid or volunteer position? Is he or she able to engage in social and recreational activities? Although the opinions of third-party payers may vary as to the importance of these issues, there is no question that PTs must ultimately understand their patient's deficits at the disability level, that is, as they affect the patient's ability to relate to society and to fulfill their life roles.

How is disability-based information best obtained? The first step is to spend *time* talking with, and listening to, patients. Although time is often limited in rehabilitation settings, PTs can prevent many missed diagnoses and develop an appropriate plan of care from the onset if they spend an adequate amount of time gathering pertinent information about their patients. Simply asking some basic questions can provide the therapist with valuable information about the problems affecting a patient's life. Indeed, asking these questions

early often saves time, because it enables the therapist to be more selective in his or her examination.

Assessment at the disability level clearly sets the rehabilitation professional apart from many other medical professionals. Medical doctors, for example, spend much of their time determining an accurate pathologic condition and relating the patient's impairments to that condition. Conversely, PTs should (and often do) spend a significant amount of their time at the other end of the disability spectrum—focusing on the interrelationship between disability and functional limitations and between functional limitations and impairments. Obtaining disability information that encompasses a patient's specific life roles provides the foundation for shaping the rehabilitation process. As noted in Chapter 1, it is the starting point for the process of rehabilitation.

DOCUMENTING ELEMENTS OF DISABILITY

The *Guide to Physical Therapist Practice* outlines various aspects of patient/client history taking that are part of the examination process; several of these are pertinent to disability documentation. Specifically, *general health status, employment/work, functional status and activity level, living environment, social history,* and *social/health habits* each encompass disability and social history information. These have been compressed into three major categories for simplification of documentation: (1) home environment, (2) employment/work, and (3) health status (Figure 5-1). The degree to which each of these headings is used may differ depending on the institution and patient population. Case Examples 5-1, 5-2, and 5-3 provide sample documentation of disability and social history in different clinical settings.

The *focus* of disability documentation varies for different patients and in different settings. Certainly, the primary concern for patients who are very sick in the hospital is working toward attainment of an independent functional status, such as their ability to dress themselves and shower. In fact, in a *hospital setting*, documentation of a patient's work status, home environment, and health status often refers to what the patient was doing *before* being admitted to the hospital (What was his or her job? What sports and recreational activities did he or she enjoy participating in?). When the patient is receiving *outpatient* or *home-based services*, the focus of documentation should reflect current disability issues (Is the patient currently working, and if so, at what functional level?; Can he or she return to recreational sports?).

Elements of Disability

Home Environment   The PT documents a wide range of information pertaining to the patient's home and living situation under this heading, often including details about the type of home, the number of floors, and the number and type of stairs. If a patient uses certain medical equipment, such as a wheelchair or a raised toilet seat, this is reported here. The PT should describe the equipment and how it is used in sufficient detail. For example: "Pt. uses a lightweight wheelchair, with gel cushion and swing-away leg rests, for mobility within the home."

Description of the patient's family and caregiver resources are also components of the home environment. Cultural beliefs and behaviors, as they are relevant to the rehabilitation process, should also be included in this section. However, specific details about a patient's personal life that are not pertinent to his or her current medical condition or reason for referral should not be included in patient documentation. For example, it would rarely be necessary to refer to a patient as "divorced," or to identify a person's specific religious affiliation.

Employment/Work   If a patient or client is working or has recently stopped working because of an injury or illness, the nature of the work should be documented

---

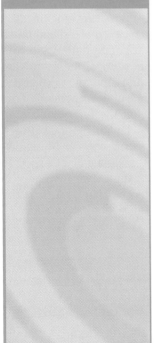

CASE EXAMPLE 5-1	**Documenting Disability and Social History**

Setting: Inpatient acute care

Name: Lisa Jeter   *D.O.B.:* 5/20/49   *DATE OF EVAL:* 12/10/00

Current Condition: s/p L middle cerebral artery stroke, 1215/00

DISABILITY/SOCIAL HISTORY

Home Environment: Pt. lives c̄ her husband and 2 teenage children in 2-story home; 5 steps to enter c̄ 2 railings and 12 steps to 2nd floor with 1 railing (on R to ↑). Bedrooms and bathroom are on 2nd floor. Pt's. husband works full-time, and states that he would need additional support to assist in pt's. daily care skills if she is not independent when she returns home.

Employment/Work: Pt. employed as a data analyst; works out of her home 4 days/wk. using computer, fax machine, and telephone.

Health Status: Before stroke, pt. and her husband split daily household duties. Pt. was responsible for the family's money management, laundry, cooking, and shopping. Pt. led an active lifestyle—enjoyed jogging every morning with her daughter; actively coached daughter's soccer team, and her husband reports her health as being excellent. Previous recreational activities include camping trips, skiing, and going to the theatre.

COMPONENTS OF DOCUMENTING REASON FOR REFERRAL: DISABILITY AND SOCIAL HISTORY

Home environment
- Living environment and community characteristics
- Family and living situation
- Family and caregiver resources
- Devices and equipment (e.g. assistive, adaptive, orthotic, protective, supportive, prosthetic)
- Projected discharge destination
- Cultural beliefs and behaviors

Employment/work (job/school/play)
- Current and prior work (job/school/play)

Health status (self-report, family report, caregiver report)
- Prior functional status in self-care and home management, including activities of daily living (ADL) and instrumental activities of daily living (IADL)
- Community, leisure, and social activity participation
- General health perception/quality of life
- Physical function (e.g., mobility, sleep patterns, restricted bed days)
- Psychological function (e.g., memory, reasoning ability, depression, anxiety)
- Behavioral health risks (e.g., smoking, drug abuse)
- Level of physical fitness

FIGURE 5-1

Components of documenting reasons for referral: disability and social history. This figure attempts to incorporate terminology found in the *Guide to Physical Therapist Practice*, 2001, p. S36.

in sufficient detail. Such notations typically include a listing or description of the tasks or activities the patient performs in a typical day (e.g., typing, writing, lifting), and any unique requirements to the patient's job (e.g., "lifting > 50 lbs," "standing for > 1 hr at a time"). The therapist should also document here any volunteer work in which the patient is or was participating (e.g., "volunteers at hospital transporting patients 1 ×/wk").

Health Status   In this category the therapist provides information pertaining to the patient's overall health and wellness. This information could include physical and psychological functioning, level of fitness, and behavioral health risks. Measurement of health status also encompasses participation in community, leisure, and social activities, which are essential to an individual's quality of life. Providing accurate and reasonable

documentation about a person's inability to participate in these activities is critical to justifying services for many patients who may appear "high functioning." For example, simply documenting that the "pt. enjoys socializing" does not provide information that is sufficiently detailed to design an appropriate intervention plan aimed at minimizing the patient's disability. The PT could instead state that the "pt. enjoys playing bridge 1 ×/wk at the neighborhood senior center and going out to dinner 2 ×/month at local restaurants".

It is important to contrast *current* level of functioning and participation with *prior* level of functioning and participation. *Prior functional status* refers to the degree of functional skill of a patient in self-care, leisure, and social activities before the onset of the current medical diagnosis or problem. Determination of prior functional status is particularly relevant for older patients or those with previous medical conditions. Such patients may not have been independent in all activities before the onset of their current condition; they may have had some limitations as a result of other medical conditions or problems related to their current medical condition. For example, a patient who has had a stroke may have had a pre-existing condition of emphysema. This may have limited the patient's walking distance, secondary to pulmonary limitations, even before having the stroke.

The goal of therapy is often to restore the patient to at least the level of prior functioning. Sometimes the goal is to restore the patient to a higher level of functioning, as in the case of a patient with arthritis who elects to have a total knee replacement. Because that patient's functional abilities may have been significantly limited by the arthritis, the knee replacement may enable the patient to improve to a significantly higher functional level.

SPECIFICITY OF DOCUMENTATION

Information about a person's home situation, employment status, and leisure activities should be sufficiently detailed so that it is useful to the therapist or other personnel reading the report. The information presented in this section helps to shape both the patient's prognosis and the intervention plan. Furthermore, it provides the foundation for developing appropriate and realistic goals that will be based on the patient's current level of disability and his or her lifestyle.

An example could be a patient who has had a recent heart attack and is undergoing cardiac rehabilitation. It would not be sufficient to document "Pt. led an active lifestyle before heart attack." If a goal of the patient is to return to this active lifestyle, documentation of the details of these activities is important. This information might instead be documented as: "Before heart attack, pt. ran 4 miles 4 ×/wk and enjoyed sailing his sailboat 1-2 ×/wk in the summer." Case Examples 5-1, 5-2, and 5-3 further illustrate this point.

MEASUREMENT OF DISABILITY

A person's disability refers to any limitations in his or her ability to accomplish personal or societal roles. Such limitations can be measured in different ways, including the following:

PREVENTING DISABILITY

In some therapist-patient encounters there is no clear disability. The most obvious example is primary prevention, in which the patient is a healthy individual with only the risk of developing a disabling illness. In addition, therapists often see patients in the acute stages of an illness or immediately after injury, when a clear disability has not yet developed. Indeed, in such instances the therapist actively intervenes to prevent disability from occurring (secondary prevention) or limit its severity (tertiary prevention). For example, a patient who sees a PT for acute low back pain is at risk for developing chronic low back syndrome, which might lead to loss of employment or inability to fulfill other roles. An athlete with a tendon injury might need carefully controlled rest and stabilization to prevent long-term loss of the ability to participate in competitive sports. A newborn with spina bifida may exhibit little current disability but is clearly at risk for future disability; early intervention is designed to minimize future disability.

The examples cited in the preceding paragraph point to the need for a slightly modified concept of top-down rehabilitation, but one in which the patient's disability (the roles that the patient is unable to fulfill) still plays a dominant role in determining the rehabilitation plan. We therefore introduce a concept referred to as *potential disability*, which involves identifying the life roles in which the patient might lose function. As in the traditional use of the term *disability*, considering potential disabilities helps PTs to focus their goals and intervention plan. A patient with acute low back pain is used as an example. If the potential disability were occupational in nature, intervention might be focused on teaching the patient to perform certain work-related skills safely and alternative ways to accomplish certain tasks. If, however, the potential disability were in competitive athletics, a very different approach would be used—one with greater emphasis on strengthening muscles and fine-tuning movement strategies so that the patient could continue to perform at a high level without causing further injury.

Clinicians can use a considerable database of evidence to identify potential disability. Numerous studies have shown that the natural history of certain diseases (and risk factors) lead to predictable disabilities (Incalzi et al., 1992; Adams et al., 1999; Curtis & Black, 1999; Feuerstein et al., 1999; Stuck et al., 1999; Lamb et al., 2000; Westhoff et al., 2000). Clinicians can use this evidence to determine whether a significant risk of future disability exists and justify intervention on that basis.

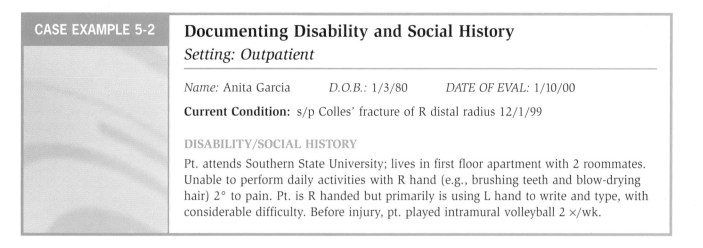

CASE EXAMPLE 5-2

Documenting Disability and Social History
Setting: Outpatient

Name: Anita Garcia   *D.O.B.:* 1/3/80   *DATE OF EVAL:* 1/10/00

Current Condition: s/p Colles' fracture of R distal radius 12/1/99

DISABILITY/SOCIAL HISTORY

Pt. attends Southern State University; lives in first floor apartment with 2 roommates. Unable to perform daily activities with R hand (e.g., brushing teeth and blow-drying hair) 2° to pain. Pt. is R handed but primarily is using L hand to write and type, with considerable difficulty. Before injury, pt. played intramural volleyball 2 ×/wk.

- Caregiver burden/level of assistance. Does a person need assistance from caregivers to complete activities important to daily functioning?
- Quality of life. How is a person's quality of life affected or changed by the current condition? What is the person's *overall level of participation* in various activities that are important for his or her daily life roles?

Caregiver burden/level of assistance measures the amount of assistance from another person that is needed for an individual to perform certain tasks related to specific roles. Level of assistance for any one particular skill, such as dressing, bathing, or walking, is typically documented as part of *Functional Status.* However, whether or not assistance is needed for a range of activities is an important global measure of disability. For example, documenting the need for a personal aide to assist with morning activities of daily living (ADLs) is an example of caregiver burden. The next chapter outlines ways to document level of assistance for specific functional skills.

Some patients may not require assistance to accomplish a certain role, but they have difficulty fulfilling that role to the degree they once could (e.g., continuing to work at a job even though unable to perform certain heavy lifting tasks). This difficulty would affect that person's *quality of life.* Alternatively, an individual may be unable to perform specific activities at all, regardless of assistance (e.g., many recreational activities, such as playing golf). This too would affect an individual's quality of life. Specifically, *quality of life* describes to what degree any limitation in *participation* of activities related to life roles affects the enjoyment or sense of satisfaction that a person experiences in a domain that is important to that person.

Documentation of disability assumes a different form in pediatric settings. Those activities applicable to an

adult may not be appropriate for a child. For example, the Pediatric Evaluation of Disability Inventory (PEDI) was developed specifically to address the lack of appropriate disability-based tools in the pediatric population (Haley et al., 1992). This instrument was designed to measure caregiver burden and functional skills for activities meaningful to a child's life and independent functioning.

Obtaining Disability Information

Disability-based information can be gathered in several ways: interview, questionnaire, and direct observation.

Interview   The therapist can begin the disability inquiry by asking the patient some simple questions (Table 5-1). Specifically, the therapist needs to ascertain the patient's *premorbid lifestyle* and the *patient's current goals* for regaining that lifestyle. The interview can be conducted with either the patient, or a caregiver, or both. For young children, interviews are often conducted with the parent.

Table 5-1 lists various questions that could be asked to ascertain disability level information. The type of questions asked during a disability interview should vary depending on the age and medical diagnosis of the patient.

Questionnaires and Patient Self-Report   Although conducting a basic interview often is the quickest way to obtain disability information, the use of standardized assessment tools can provide more reliable and systematic measure of disability. Table 5-2 outlines some of the common standardized tools to measure disability. The tools listed primarily measure quality of life obtained by patient self-report. Self-report is a very important piece of an examination, particularly in assessment of outcomes. Patients sometimes have little or no improvement in impairments or even in particular functional abilities, but they may have significantly improved their quality of life. For example, they may have developed strategies of coping with pain or effective compensatory strategies to accomplish tasks. Alternatively, they may show improvement in impairments, such as weakness or limited ROM, with no corresponding reduction of disability. Patient self-report is almost always the primary source of information about changes in disability status.

Self-report measures are often thought to be less valuable because they are not "objective." Self-report measures are inherently subjective, and this subjectivity increases the chance that the patient will provide inaccurate or exaggerated information. Some information, nevertheless, is best obtained through self-report. For example, the Oswestry Disability Questionnaire (Roland and Jenner, 1989) evaluates a patient's perceived limitations in various life activities. Such limitations often are difficult to ascertain by physical examination, in part because they measure activities that are not readily evaluated in a clinic setting (e.g., sleeping and traveling).

For documentation purposes, only the scores from standardized tests should be reported in the body of an evaluation report. The therapist may choose to summarize components from the test that are pertinent or provide a brief interpretation of the test results. This applies to all forms of standardized testing, including those used for function and impairments (see Chapters 6 and 7). The completed standardized test form should be included in the patient's record, although third-party payers may not see it. Often third-party payers see only an evaluation report or summary.

Direct Observation Disability-based examinations may also be conducted through direct observation. The

TABLE 5-1	SAMPLE INTERVIEW QUESTIONS TO ASCERTAIN DISABILITY-BASED INFORMATION	
	Young Child	**Older Man**
Patient	5 y.o. boy with cerebral palsy, lives at home with parents (interview directed at parent)	64 y.o. semi-retired carpenter, with rotator cuff tear, divorced, lives alone, has 2 grandchildren
Home environment	• Describe your child's home and living situation. • Do you have any stairs? How many? • Does your child have any siblings? • Who else provides care for your child?	• Describe your home and living situation. • Do you have any stairs? How many? • Do your children live close by? • Are they able to assist you in any way with household tasks?
Occupational/work	• Is your child able to participate fully in all school activities, including sitting at his desk during lesson plans, and participating in gym class?	• To what extent have you recently been involved in your work as a carpenter? • To what degree are you limited in your ability to work?
Health status	• How would you describe your child's overall health? • What types of play or recreational activities does your child engage in? • Does he have any difficulties or limitations in activities he would like to engage in, but is unable? • Does your child participate in age-appropriate chores in the house, such as helping to clean his room? • What types of social interactions does your child engage in? Does your child have any difficulty engaging in play with his peers?	• How would you describe you overall health? • Are you able to maintain the basic upkeep of your apartment, for example, doing the cleaning or the laundry? • Has your social activity (for example, time spent with family and friends) changed at all because of your current condition? • What recreational activities (e.g., sports, leisure activities) did you engage in prior to this recent injury? Are you having any difficulty or limitations performing those activities now?

Functional Independence Measure (FIM) (Keith et al., 1987) and Barthel Index (Collin et al., 1988) require the use of direct observation to describe functional skill levels (see Table 5-2). Because these levels are based largely on the degree of caregiver assistance, the FIM and Barthel Index (among others) should properly be categorized as measures of disability. However, many health care professionals and agencies consider these

TABLE 5-2   A LIST OF SOME COMMONLY USED STANDARDIZED MEASURES OF DISABILITY*

	Population	Purpose
QUESTIONNAIRES/ SELF-REPORT		
Pediatric Evaluation of Disability Inventory (PEDI) (Haley et al., 1992)	Young children age 6 months-7.5 years	Designed to measure basic functional abilities, amount of caregiver burden and adaptive devices needed to accomplish mobility, self-care and social activities; provides age-related normative scores
SF-36 (Stewart et al., 1988)	General adult population	Includes 36 items pertaining to general well being, and frequency and degree of participation in daily living, social and recreational activities
Sickness Impact Profile (Bergner et al., 1981; van Straten et al, 1997)	General adult population; adapted version for stroke population	Self-report measure of health status on 12 subscales
Oswestry Disability Questionnaire (Fairbank et al., 1980)	Individuals with low back or neck pain	Self-report measure that results in an index of a patient's perceived disability based on 10 functional areas
Rheumatoid Hand Disability Scale (Duruoz, 1996)	Adults with rheumatoid arthritis	Measure of functional hand disability; includes 18 hand activity questions with 6 levels of answers
Lower Extremity Activity Profile (Finch and Kennedy, 1995)	Individuals undergoing knee replacement surgery	Measures client's satisfaction and perception of difficulty during self care, mobility, household activities, work, leisure, and social activities
LEVEL OF ASSISTANCE/ DIRECT OBSERVATION		
Barthel Index (Mahoney and Barthel, 1968)†	Rehabilitation—stroke, brain injury	Determines *level of assistance* in various ADLs; widely used in studies of stroke outcome
Functional Independence Measure (FIM) (Keith et al., 1987)†	Rehabilitation—stroke, brain injury, orthopedic conditions	Developed out of the need to establish a reliable, uniform method of classifying rehabilitation patients to measure outcomes; measures *level of assistance* in 6 functional areas

*Refer to references listed to determine each measure's proper use and measurement properties.
†Note that the Barthel Index and the FIM, while global measures of disability, also measure level of assistance on specific functional skills.

CASE EXAMPLE 5-3	**Documenting Disability and Social History**

Setting: Outpatient

Name: Joe Smith   D.O.B.: 1/10/52   *DATE OF EVAL:* 7/14/99

Current Condition: L4-5 disc herniation, onset of symptoms 7/2/99

DISABILITY/SOCIAL HISTORY

Home environment: Pt. lives at home with his wife and 2 young daughters in a 2-story house (bedrooms on second floor). Pt.'s wife works full-time.

Employment/work: Pt. works as an independent building contractor. He is currently doing paper work at his desk and making phone calls but has not yet returned to any physical labor. Job entails 60% moderate-heavy lifting (up to 100 lbs) and 40% desk work, requiring sitting at desk and phone for 1-2 hrs at a time.

Health Status: Oswestry Disability Questionnaire 28/50 (indicating severe disability). He is currently unable to perform daily household duties (e.g., cleaning, taking out trash) 2° to pain. Before onset of LBP 2 mos ago, pt. led relatively inactive lifestyle. Enjoyed watching sports on television; currently able to sit for only 30 min at a time to watch TV. Previously enjoyed attending daughter's softball games; has not attended a game since surgery due to inability to sit on bleacher-style seats. Pt. also enjoyed going to movies and to dinner with wife; he has not attempted either, due to inability to sit for more than 30 min. Hx of smoking 1 pack/day for past 20 yrs.

---

to be functional measures. This conflict illustrates the difficulty that can arise in making a clear distinction between the concepts of *functional dependence* and *disability.*

Nonstandardized measures of disability also may involve observing the patient in a natural setting. For example, in the home care setting the therapist might observe a patient performing the range of skills that encompass his or her ability to be a homemaker. A common example of disability-based evaluations, as well as an area of specialty practice in physical therapy, is on-site work evaluations. A therapist can provide accurate disability-based examinations that ultimately are most meaningful to the therapist and the patients by directly observing patients in their work environment and their specific difficulties in performing certain tasks.

SUMMARY

- Documentation at the *disability level* addresses the ability of a patient to perform the specific roles pertinent to his or her everyday life.

- Disability documentation is categorized by home environment, work/occupation, and health status.

- Disability is specific to an individual and his or her environment. In a pediatric setting, disability is often related to a child's ability to play or attend school. For an adult patient, disability encompasses the ability to perform specific functions related to daily care, work/occupation, social life, and leisure.

- Limitations in participation of various life roles can be measured by caregiver burden/level of assistance and quality of life.

- Disability information is most commonly obtained through patient and family interviews and from the medical record. Through the interview process the therapist ascertains the patient's *premorbid lifestyle* and determine the *patient's current goals* for regaining that lifestyle.

- Standardized questionnaires use self-reporting to determine a patient's overall health status and participation in recreational, social, occupational, and personal activities.

EXERCISE 5-1

Identify the errors in the following statements documenting Reason for Referral: Disability and Social History. Errors could include not enough detail; irrelevant information, negative connotation, and labeling; or inappropriate for this section. Indicate the specific word or words that are problematic, if applicable. Rewrite a more appropriate statement in the space provided.

Statement	What is Wrong?	Rewrite Statement
EXAMPLE: Pt. cannot return home.	Not enough detail about what specific situation prevents the patient from returning home.	Pt. cannot return home at the present time. There are 2 flights of stairs leading to her apartment, and no modifications can be made.
1. Able to walk 50 feet with straight cane.		
2. Needs help with some activities.		
3. Pt. is a T12 paraplegic who is confined to a wheelchair.		
4. Has poor motivation to return to work.		
5. Works on a loading dock.		
6. TBI patient requires A c̄ all ADLs.		
7. Patient enjoys outdoor sports.		
8. Pt. complains that she cannot return to work 2° to architectural barriers.		

Statement	What is Wrong?	Rewrite Statement
9. Pt. will return to work in full capacity in 8 weeks.		
10. Pt. was very active before her injury.		
11. Suzie's mother reports she doesn't go on any play dates.		
12. Pt. is in poor shape.		
13. Pt. lives in an apartment.		
14. Pt. has a history of bad health habits.		
15. Pt. uses adaptive equipment.		

EXERCISE 5-2

The following statements are taken from various sections of an initial evaluation report in an outpatient setting. Extract the information that would be appropriate to include in this section of the report (Reason for Referral: Disability/Social History). Indicate those statements that do not belong in this section. Rewrite this information under the appropriate subheadings in the space provided below. The sentences should flow together smoothly.

1. Pt. underwent L transtibial amputation on 6/18/99 at County Hospital and is now referred for physical therapy evaluation.

2. Pt. lives with her daughter in an apartment building on the 2nd floor. There is an elevator that sometimes doesn't work.

3. Pt. has a raised toilet seat, grab bars, and shower chair in shower.

4. Pt. needs assistance from daughter every other morning for bathing.

5. Pt. is able to dress her upper body with setup but requires increased time, verbal cues, and some help to do pants and shoes.

6. Pt. enjoys watching Jeopardy and Wheel of Fortune every evening.

7. Pt. is not currently working 2° to walking and standing limitations.

8. Before surgery, pt. enjoyed 2-3 outings per month to mall or to visit friends.

9. Pt. will be independent in outdoor ambulation for distances >1000 ft without assistive device.

10. Before surgery, pt. was working 3 days/wk as a retail sales clerk, which required standing and walking most of the day.

11. Pt. has a hx of IDDM × 10 yrs; HTN × 5 yrs.

12. Pt. reports leading a relatively sedentary lifestyle, and does not participate in regular exercise program.

Home environment: _____

_____

_____

Occupation/work: _____

_____

_____

Health status: _____

_____

_____

Statements that do not belong in this section (statement numbers): _____

_____

_____

EXERCISE 5-3

This exercise is designed to practice patient-interview techniques for obtaining disability and social history information. Students should form groups of pairs. The Answer Key in the back of the book contains two case reports (A and B) documenting disability information. One student (acting as patient) should carefully read Case Report A. The second student (acting as therapist) will ask the patient questions aimed at obtaining a comprehensive disability assessment. The patient should be careful to answer directly only those questions asked by the therapist. Then students should switch roles for Case Report B. The therapist may choose to record answers on a separate sheet of paper and write the final documentation in the space provided.

CASE REPORT A	*Setting: Outpatient*

Name: Terry O'Connor   *D.O.B.:* 3/23/33   *DATE OF EVAL:* 7/2/99

REASON FOR REFERRAL

Current Condition: Right hip bursitis, onset around 5/10/99. Pt. is a 66-year-old female who had a gradual onset of pain approximately 2 months ago in her right thigh, which progressed to a continuous "throbbing pain." Pain radiates from the right hip to the right knee. Pt. does not attribute it to any particular incident.

Home Environment

Occupation/Work

Health Status

CASE REPORT B

Setting: Inpatient Rehabilitation

Name: Tommy Jones *D.O.B.:* 5/12/79 *DATE OF EVAL:* 7/2/99 *Admission date:* 7/2/99

REASON FOR REFERRAL

Current Condition: C7 incomplete SCI 2° to MVA on 6/15/99. Pt. was transferred this morning from County Acute Care Hospital, where he has been since his accident. Medical records reveal one episode of orthostatic hypotension on coming to sitting and two episodes of autonomic dysreflexia. Pt. underwent surgery on 6/16/99 for anterior cervical fusion. Currently cleared for all rehabilitation activities per Dr. Johnston (per phone conversation this morning).

Home Environment

Occupation/Work

Health Status

---

*Note: Patient is in a hospital setting, so disability/social history information will be based mainly on patient's abilities and activities before admission to hospital.

CHAPTER 6

Documenting Functional Status: A Skill-Based Model

LEARNING OBJECTIVES

After reading this chapter and completing the exercises, the reader will be able to:

1. Define function and functional limitations.
2. Describe the categories in *The Guide's* tests and measures that relate to functional status.
3. Discuss the factors involved in deciding which functional abilities should be included in documentation.
4. Identify and classify various aspects of documenting a patient or client's functional status.
5. Appropriately categorize activities of daily living and instrumental activities of daily living for documentation purposes.
6. Document functional activities using a skill-based framework.

DEFINING AND CATEGORIZING FUNCTIONS

A *function* is defined as "the action for which a person is fitted or employed" (Davies, 2000). According to the Nagi model, a *functional limitation* refers to "limitation in performance at the level of the whole organism or person" (Nagi, 1965). If an action is to be considered functional in nature, it must (1) be meaningful to an individual, and (2) help an individual to fulfill his or her roles (e.g., spouse, parent, volunteer, worker, student, pet owner).

Although the term *functional limitations* is used in the Nagi model of disablement, other terms such as *functional status* or *functional abilities* are probably better suited for documentation purposes. The term *functional limitations* has a negative connotation and suggests that only limitations in function are considered. In most cases, documentation should include abilities *and* limitations as they relate to function. In this book the term *functional status* is used as a global category for documenting skills, abilities, and limitations related to function.

Six of the 24 groupings in the list of tests and measures presented in the *Guide to Physical Therapist Practice* have components that measure functional abilities:

- Aerobic capacity and endurance
- Environmental, home, and work (job/school/play) barriers
- Gait, locomotion, and balance
- Neuromotor development and sensory integration
- Self-care and home management (including activities of daily living [ADLs] and instrumental activities of daily living [IADLs])
- Work (job/school/play), community, and leisure integration or reintegration (including IADLs)

Chapter 2 of the *Guide* provides a detailed list of tests and measures under each of these groupings. However, the *Guide* does not organize tests and measures according to impairment and function. Indeed, sometimes the differentiation is difficult, as in the case of "gait, locomotion, and balance." The task of walking is certainly a function, but describing the details of the gait pattern or the balance needed to maintain walking is more closely related to impairments. In fact, the differentiation between impairments and functional skills may be considered as a continuum rather than a strict separation. Figure 6-1 and the Box on the opposite page illustrate this concept.

Functional status is arguably the most important component of physical therapy documentation. Functional information is used to justify the need for physical therapy services, as well as to show improvement over time. Pathologic conditions and the resulting impairments are important insofar as they affect a patient's daily functioning. Functional activities are those that are meaningful to patients: can they walk, run, get dressed, reach, and grasp for objects? Improvements in these activities should be a primary outcome of physical therapy intervention. Case Examples 6-1, 6-2, and 6-3 provide sample documentation of functional status in different clinical settings.

DOCUMENTING TASK PERFORMANCE

Physical therapy intervention often entails practice of specific tasks, such as walking, squatting, lifting, reaching, and grasping. In effect, these tasks are actions that are used in a wide range of functional activities. Therapists often quantify and qualify performance on tasks as a measure of a patient's functional ability.

Reaching, grasping, walking, and many other types of movement patterns are *elements* of functional activities; they are not functional activities per se. They are not considered functional because they do not have a clearly definable and meaningful goal or purpose. For instance, gait evaluation describes the *movement patterns* used for walking. Gait deviations (e.g., Trendelenburg, excessive circumduction, foot drop) are therefore impair-

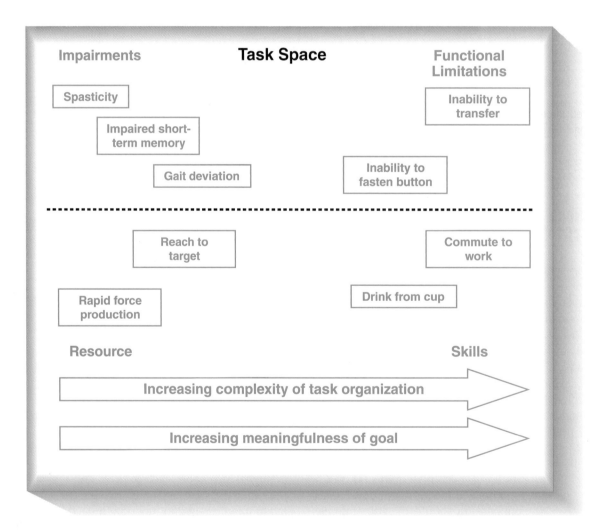

FIGURE 6-1

The task space represents the interface between impairments and functional limitations, or skills and resources. Tasks can have stronger components of either function/skills or impairment/resources depending on the nature and goal of the task.

THE GRAY LINE BETWEEN FUNCTIONS AND IMPAIRMENTS

As mentioned in Chapter 1, the Nagi model affords different perspectives to describe physical therapy patients and their conditions. A patient's condition can be described in terms of the pathology, impairments, functional limitations, or disabilities. These are not separate and distinct characteristics of the patient; they are all aspects of the same disabling condition, described in different measurement systems. Furthermore, some overlap occurs between levels of the Nagi model. For example, the classification of an evaluation finding as an impairment versus a functional limitation is often a slightly gray area.

The crucial distinction between impairments and functional limitations is between means and ends. Functions are activities described in terms of goals or ends. The impairment level describes means to an end: by what mechanisms the goal is accomplished. This important distinction can be illustrated with reference to two movement systems: balance and walking.

BALANCE

Balance is a perfect example of a characteristic that is difficult to categorize. Balance in its purest sense is described at the impairment level, reflecting the ability of an individual to maintain an upright position against gravity. However, balance is often evaluated through a set of tasks that might be considered "functional." For example, the ability to stand in one place for more than 30 sec is certainly functional, as is the ability to reach to the floor to pick up an object. Thus, if balance is described in terms of the goal, it is a function. If it is analyzed in terms of the component mechanisms (e.g., increased sway, role of vision), then it is at the impairment level.

WALKING

Walking is another example of a task that combines both impairments and functional limitations. Therapists often describe walking in functional terms—how long a patient can walk, how quickly, with how much assistance. However, another important component of walking is evaluation of *how* a person walks—his or her gait pattern. Gait analysis can be considered a measure at the impairment level. Therapists often describe gait deviations (such as a Trendelenburg gait) that reflect the presence of an underlying impairment (gluteus medius weakness). Again, if the walking is measured in terms of goal attainment (e.g., distance, speed), then it is a function. If gait is analyzed in terms of why the goal is *not* being achieved (e.g., insufficient knee flexion during swing or inadequate stance phase control of knee extensors), then walking is being described in terms of impairments.

CLASSIFICATION

Even more problems arise in classification of standardized tests and measures. Standardized tests sometime measure across different levels of the disablement model (e.g., measuring some components of function and some of impairments). This in fact may be desirable in situations in which a global standardized test is needed.

These difficulties with classification and distinction may seem academic, but documentation can be frustrating if therapists are searching for clear-cut answers (e.g., Is balance a function or an impairment?). The following strategy is suggested. All information about a topic (e.g., standing ability, balance control) should be included under one subheading (e.g., standing balance). Even if a particular topic mixes function and impairments, cohesive presentation of that information in the written report is important (see Case Example 6-1). Reading a report with information about a single component scattered throughout the report is difficult. Whether the information is categorized under "function" or "impairments" can depend on the focus of information being written.

ments. Walking to the bathroom or walking outside on grass to get through a yard describe *functions,* because they have a meaningful goal. As stated earlier, functions are actions that are meaningful to an individual and help an individual to fulfill his or her roles in life. However, in certain situations, documentation of a patient's performance of tasks outside the context of specific functional skills may be useful. For example, a therapist could document a person's ability to reach forward into space, or to take steps in the parallel bars. For documentation purposes, such elemental tasks are most logically reported in the Functional Status section of the report.

Elemental tasks represent the interface between functional limitations and impairments (see Figure 6-1). Evaluation of the movement patterns and strategies used to perform such tasks provides important insight to the underlying impairments that affect function. This allows a broader analysis of task performance beyond the specific functional skill of which the task is a component. Task evaluation may bridge many functional skills. For example, the ability to squat is important for functional skills ranging from using the bathroom to picking up an object. Importantly, therapists may use task analysis to derive a deeper understanding of the contribution of various impairments to functional performance. Documentation of elemental tasks, therefore, often includes information about how the movement was performed and the effect of any impairments on functional performance.

Although evaluation of task performance is an important aspect of the physical therapy evaluation process, therapists should give priority to context-based functional assessment. For example, tasks such as reaching

Documenting Functional Status

Setting: Homecare

Name: Maureen Smith   *D.O.B.:* 5/12/38   *DATE OF EVALUATION:* 7/3/99

Current Condition: 61 y.o. woman had L side cerebral hemorrhage 5/14/99 with resulting R-sided hemiparesis; discharged from Rehab Center on 7/1/99 where she spent 4 wks after acute care stay at Community Hospital.

CURRENT FUNCTIONAL STATUS

Bed Mobility: Pt. rolls to R I'ly; rolls to L c̄ min A to bring R leg over. Needs mod A to position self in bed c̄ use of trapeze.

Sitting Ability: *On bed:* Bed needs to be positioned so pt.'s feet are flat on floor. Able to sit for 10 min (limited due to fatigue) independently. Unable to reach > 1″ outside arm's length in all directions. *In wheelchair:* Can sit I'ly in W/C. After about 30 min pt. begins to lean to R side and cannot straighten self s̄ A.

Standing Ability: Requires mod A to stand for 20 sec c̄ R AFO.

W/C Transfer ↔ Bed: Uses SB to transfer from bed to wheelchair (toward the left side only) and back with min A to set up SB and begin initial movement on board. Completes task in approx. 1 min.

Mobility in Home: Pt. uses W/C as primary means of mobility in home. Can propel W/C with one-arm drive in home, except into bathroom (too narrow). Outside mobility limited to propulsion on level surfaces for 5 min, c̄ HR ↑ to 110 bpm. Requires A to negotiate curbs, ramps, and uneven terrain.

Feeding: Pt. needs A to set up plate, utensils, and cup but can eat with spoon or fork with L hand. Uses modified scoop-plate to get food onto utensil. Needs A to cut foods. Can drink using a light cup or with a straw. Self-care, grooming, and bathroom transfers: Refer to OT eval.

---

and grasping often can be assessed within the context of a functional activity, such as eating or brushing teeth. A person's ability to perform reaching and grasping behaviors is affected by the context in which they are performed (e.g., in a sitting or standing position). Similarly, assessment of gait abnormalities may differ depending on the context in which walking occurs (e.g., walking on tile versus carpeting).

DOCUMENTING PERFORMANCE OF FUNCTIONAL ACTIVITIES

One of the important roles of a physical therapist is to determine *which* functional activities are meaningful to a specific individual and help that person achieve independence and skill in these activities (Case Example 6-2).

Many possible functional activities could be important for an individual. Pertinent functional activities are those that are related to a person's specific life roles and relevant to the patient's therapeutic goals. Functional activities can be categorized in each of the three life roles: personal, occupational, and leisure (recreational). Some activities are common to almost everyone. For example, many activities related to fulfilling the personal life role, referred to as ADLs, are necessary for almost everyone to perform (Figure 6-2). Other activities are more specific to a person's life roles, such as those required for work or recreational sports. Figure 6-3 presents examples of common activities related to personal, occupational, and leisure roles. In this figure, ADLs are categorized as personal activities by the context or environment in which they are performed. This categorization can be helpful for organizing the section of a patient interview regarding function: begin by asking about functions that are

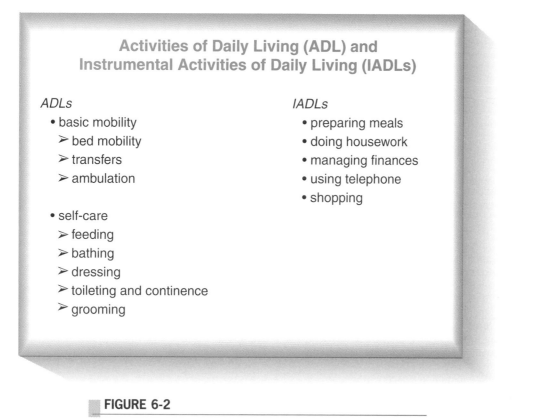

Activities of Daily Living (ADL) and Instrumental Activities of Daily Living (IADLs)

ADLs
- basic mobility
  - ➢ bed mobility
  - ➢ transfers
  - ➢ ambulation

- self-care
  - ➢ feeding
  - ➢ bathing
  - ➢ dressing
  - ➢ toileting and continence
  - ➢ grooming

IADLs
- preparing meals
- doing housework
- managing finances
- using telephone
- shopping

FIGURE 6-2

Activities of daily living and instrumental activities of daily living.

required in the bedroom (e.g., dressing) and continue through the rest of the house.

Documentation of functional abilities should be customized to the particular setting. The focus of functional documentation for a patient who resides in a nursing home would likely be on ADLs and some leisure activities. In contrast, a therapist may perform a specific work-site evaluation for a patient; in this case the functional documentation would likely be limited to occupational activities.

PTs can create subheadings within this section of the report to better organize the information and improve readability (see Case Examples). It is often useful to group activities or tasks together (e.g., ambulation or transfers) and include all related tasks under their appropriate headings.

For most patients who reside at home or will be returning home, the therapist is responsible for evaluating those functional abilities that are pertinent to different environmental situations. Therapists must ask themselves "In what types of environments will the patient function?" Most *tasks* can be performed in many different *environments.* For instance, the task of "walking" can

occur in a controlled, closed environment, such as the physical therapy gym in a hospital. Walking also can occur in a more variable and open environment, such as walking across a busy street. Thus simply documenting the task of "walking" is not particularly meaningful if it is devoid of environmental context. Therapists must take care to assess a range of environmental contexts as they are *meaningful* to a specific patient. (See Gentile's taxonomy of tasks for more information on environmental and task classification [Gentile, 1987]).

Functional skills for children assume a slightly different meaning. Although children generally perform many of the same personal roles as adults (e.g., bathing, dressing, eating, and general mobility), their work and leisure activities clearly differ. "Play skills" encompass a child's work and leisure activities, particularly for younger children. In physical therapy, such skills are often categorized as gross motor skills. Documentation of pediatric evaluations often includes a section on gross motor skills and a separate section on self-care or self-help skills (as they are sometimes termed).

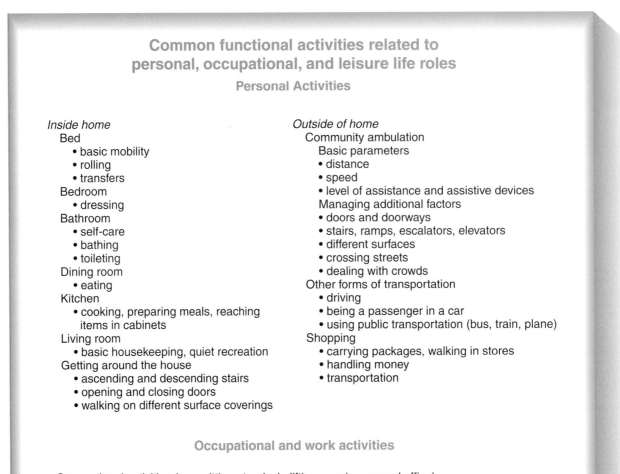

Common functional activities related to personal, occupational, and leisure life roles

Personal Activities

Inside home
Bed
- basic mobility
- rolling
- transfers

Bedroom
- dressing

Bathroom
- self-care
- bathing
- toileting

Dining room
- eating

Kitchen
- cooking, preparing meals, reaching items in cabinets

Living room
- basic housekeeping, quiet recreation

Getting around the house
- ascending and descending stairs
- opening and closing doors
- walking on different surface coverings

Outside of home
Community ambulation
Basic parameters
- distance
- speed
- level of assistance and assistive devices

Managing additional factors
- doors and doorways
- stairs, ramps, escalators, elevators
- different surfaces
- crossing streets
- dealing with crowds

Other forms of transportation
- driving
- being a passenger in a car
- using public transportation (bus, train, plane)

Shopping
- carrying packages, walking in stores
- handling money
- transportation

Occupational and work activities

- Occupational activities (e.g., sitting at a desk, lifting, moving around office)
- Work-related activities (e.g., care of others, volunteer work, community service)
- Specific educational activities (e.g., participating in class activities, moving between classrooms)
- Play activities; for children, "play" is their "work" (e.g., gross motor: ball playing, jumping, running; fine motor: doing puzzles, stacking blocks, stringing beads)

Leisure activities

- Leisure activities (e.g., going to the movies, socializing with friends)
- Recreational activities (e.g., exercising, participating in recreational sports)

FIGURE 6-3

Common function activities related to personal, occupational, and leisure life roles.

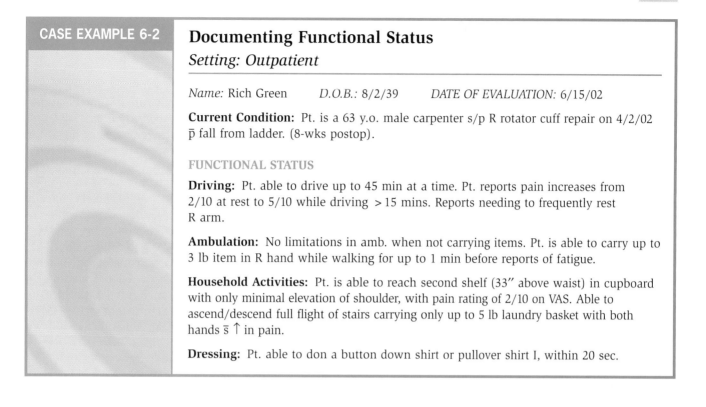

CASE EXAMPLE 6-2

Documenting Functional Status
Setting: Outpatient

Name: Rich Green   *D.O.B.:* 8/2/39   *DATE OF EVALUATION:* 6/15/02

Current Condition: Pt. is a 63 y.o. male carpenter s/p R rotator cuff repair on 4/2/02 p̄ fall from ladder. (8-wks postop).

FUNCTIONAL STATUS

Driving: Pt. able to drive up to 45 min at a time. Pt. reports pain increases from 2/10 at rest to 5/10 while driving >15 mins. Reports needing to frequently rest R arm.

Ambulation: No limitations in amb. when not carrying items. Pt. is able to carry up to 3 lb item in R hand while walking for up to 1 min before reports of fatigue.

Household Activities: Pt. is able to reach second shelf (33″ above waist) in cupboard with only minimal elevation of shoulder, with pain rating of 2/10 on VAS. Able to ascend/descend full flight of stairs carrying only up to 5 lb laundry basket with both hands s̄ ↑ in pain.

Dressing: Pt. able to don a button down shirt or pullover shirt I, within 20 sec.

Choice of Functional Activities to Document

Many possible functional limitations can be documented by the physical therapist. A patient may have limitations in ADLs, occupational and work activities, or leisure activities. How does a therapist choose which activities to document? In many situations, occupational therapists (OTs) will be involved in functional assessment, particularly for ADLs and IADLs. In such cases, PTs and OTs should collaborate and coordinate their documentation of functional abilities so as to avoid overlap.

When a PT is the only rehabilitation professional working with a patient, a very large number of functions may be relevant to the patient's care. Evaluation and documentation of all functions would be impractical and unnecessarily time consuming. In those cases, therapists must prioritize the functions that are most critical to the patient at the present time. For example, an individual who has had a severe brain injury and is just learning to sit and stand without assistance will likely be unable to perform most or all of the daily living, work, and leisure activities that he or she was able to perform before the injury. Documentation at an early point in the patient's recovery would likely focus on his or her ability to perform basic daily care skills. As the patient begins to recover from the head injury, the therapist may begin to evaluate and document different types of skills, such as those related to occupational or leisure activities. Conversely, a patient with rotator cuff tendonitis may have minimal limitations in functional abilities. The patient may be able to perform all daily living, work, and most leisure activities, and he or she may be limited only in the ability to participate in a specific recreational sport activity.

Often the purpose of documenting functional abilities is to demonstrate, at some later point, improvement in these activities over time. In many situations in which a large number of possible functional activities can be measured, therapists can choose to measure and document performance on a few activities that can be used as *benchmarks*. These activities serve as measures of progress. Therapists should carefully choose as benchmarks those activities that are most meaningful to the patient and sensitive to showing improvement as a result of intervention.

DOCUMENTATION IN THE ABSENCE OF FUNCTIONAL LIMITATIONS

When the PT documents functional status, at least a brief statement should be written if there are no limitations in certain critical skills. For example, if a person is able to perform all daily living skills independently and without any limitations, this fact should be briefly stated.

Sometimes therapists report that patients have no functional limitations, only impairments that could lead to a potential functional limitation at some later point if intervention is not provided. For patients and clients who are seen for a current medical condition (not for preventive care), it may be argued that there is, or should be, a functional limitation. If no functional limitation is present, then the therapist should question why skilled services are needed. For example, an elderly patient with lack of range of motion of the shoulder joint may be referred for physical therapy. The patient has no limitation in performing any functional activity but lacks several degrees of joint range of motion in shoulder flexion and abduction (an impairment). The therapist would be prudent to instruct the patient in range of motion and other therapeutic exercises to prevent further loss of range of motion and maintain shoulder strength. But if this impairment in range of motion does not result in functional limitations, justifying the need for extended skilled services to third-party payers may be difficult.

The important exception is a patient who receives physical therapy services with a primary goal of prevention. Many therapists provide intervention aimed at preventing disability and functional limitations. In those situations the therapist should document the *potential* disability, functional limitations, or both that may occur if the underlying pathologic condition or impairments are not addressed.

MEASUREMENT OF FUNCTIONAL PERFORMANCE: A SKILL-BASED APPROACH

Functional abilities can be measured at varying levels of complexity. The simplest measure of functional performance is *whether the goal or function was achieved.* This question can often be answered yes or no. If the goal was achieved, the next important measure is often *level of assistance*—how much assistance or what type of assistive device did the individual need to successfully complete the task? Level of assistance is typically measured by determining an estimated percentage of assistance provided by the therapist or caregiver (O'Sullivan and Schmitz, 2001). The Functional Independence Measure (FIM) is a tool used in rehabilitation settings that provides a reliable measure of level of assistance on a scale of 1 (total assistance) to 7 (complete independence; Figure 6-4). The FIM is discussed in Chapter 5 as an overall measure of disability.

Goal achievement and level of assistance provide a relatively small component in the evaluation of a person's functional abilities. In almost all cases, documentation of functional abilities should exceed simple qualitative assessment and level of independence and assess some components of skilled performance. Skill can be defined as the ability to achieve a desired outcome with *consistency, flexibility,* and *efficiency.* Table 6-1 outlines a skill-based model for evaluation of functional activities and provides examples of objective ways in which functional abilities can be documented.

CHOOSING WHICH FUNCTIONS TO MEASURE

The following guidelines should be used in deciding which functional skills should be measured and documented:

- Consider the practice setting—hospital, outpatient, home care. It will most significantly influence the PT's choice of functional skill documentation. Some agencies/hospitals mandate evaluation of specific functional skills. Collaboration with other health professionals, such as occupational therapists (OTs), will eliminate unnecessary redundancy.
- Choose activities that are meaningful to the patient, family members/caregivers, or both.
- Prioritize those functions that are most critical to the patient at this time in their rehabilitation.

- Choose *benchmark* activities—those that are amenable to showing improvement as a result of physical therapy intervention. This will differ, depending on the patient and his or her stage of learning. Simple tasks like transfers may be most useful early in rehabilitation, while more complex tasks like shopping or preparing meals are usually more appropriate later.
- If there are no limitations, include a brief statement that indicates this (e.g. "Pt. is I in all ADLs and currently reports no limitations in any functional activities"). This is generally very rare, except in the instances of intervention aimed towards prevention.

The particular aspects of a skill that a therapist chooses to measure depend on the task and the patient's level of skill. If a patient requires a high level of assistance to accomplish a task, a skill-based assessment may be limited (see Case Example 6-1). Furthermore, documentation of skill can involve any *one* or *all* of these three components: consistency, flexibility, and efficiency. For example, in early skill learning the level of assistance and consistency of performance may be more valuable measures than efficiency and flexibility. Such measures may not be meaningful until a higher level of skill is achieved.

STANDARDIZED TESTS AND MEASURES

Many different standardized tests and measures are useful in assessing functional skills. Table 6-2 lists some commonly used tests of functional performance. Several books and resources provide detailed information on the many functional assessment tools in current use, including their intended purpose (*Guide to Physical Therapist Practice*, Part 3, 2001; Cole, 1995; Lewis and McNerney, 1992; Lewis and McNerney, 1997).

Many standardized assessment tools measure across more than one level of the disablement model. For example, some tests measure both impairment and functional abilities. An example of such a test is the Berg Balance Scale (see Figure 7-1). This scale measures standing balance at the impairment level, as in standing with eyes closed or with a narrowed base of support, and at

---

FIM LEVELS

No Helper
  7 Complete Independence (Timely, Safety)
  6 Modified Independence (Device)
Helper — Modified Dependence
  5 Supervision (Subject = 100%)
  4 Minimal Assistance (Subject = 75% or more)
  3 Moderate Assistance (Subject = 50% or more)
Helper — Complete Dependence
  2 Maximal Assistance (Subject = 25% or more)
  1 Total Assistance or not testable (Subject less than 25%)

FIGURE 6-4

The Functional Independence Measure (FIM) measures level of assistance on a 7-point scale.

(Adapted from O'Sullivan and Schmitz, 2001.)

TABLE 6-1 A SKILL-BASED MODEL OF DOCUMENTING FUNCTIONAL PERFORMANCE

Skill Component	Definition	Examples	Documentation Example
Consistency	Ability to successfully perform a skill repeatedly over multiple trials or days	• Rate of goal achievement (# of successes/# of attempts) • Number of days/week able to perform • Accuracy (spatial measures of errors) • Accuracy (# of errors)	*Patient is able to transfer from bed to wheelchair using sliding board 3 out of 5 mornings with assistance of husband only for set-up.*
Flexibility	Ability to perform a skill under a variety of environmental conditions	• Height, surface, position of equipment/objects • Environment (e.g., open versus closed) • Ability to do two tasks at once	*Patient walks up 6 steps in home (8″ high) with railing; unable to carry anything in hands. Requires verbal reminders for foot placement to walk up 4 outside steps (10″ high) with railing.*
Efficiency	Ability to perform a skill within a certain level of energy expenditure (cardiovascular and musculoskeletal)	• Time to complete task • Distance completed • Speed of movement • Heart rate, respiratory rate, or blood pressure changes	*Patient can walk from bed into bathroom (10 ft) in 14.2 seconds (average time/3 trials), with increase in HR to 100 bpm*

the functional level, as in picking up an object from the floor. The tests and measures presented in Table 6-2 primarily measure performance in functional activities but may have components of disability or impairment assessments or both.

Standardized functional measures are an important aspect of physical therapy documentation; however, they should never be used *in place of* an evaluation tailored to the specific activities pertinent to a patient. If a standardized test is conducted as part of an evaluation, the therapist should report summary scores in the evaluation report and attach the scoring form to the report. Reporting results of the entire test as part of the body of an evaluation report is too cumbersome, but therapists may choose to highlight specific components or provide a brief summary of the patient's performance on the test (Case Example 6-3).

TABLE 6-2 A LIST OF SOME COMMONLY USED STANDARDIZED MEASURES OF FUNCTIONAL SKILLS*		
	Population	**Purpose**
Jebsen test of hand function (Jebsen et al., 1969)	• Orthopedic-hand and upper extremity impairments	• Timed pegboard test with norms established; primarily manipulation and also reaching
3- or 6- minute walk test (Guyatt et al., 1985)	• Cardiac, adult neurologic	• Timed walking for 3 or 6 minutes • Determine distance traveled and walking velocity and cardiovascular measures
Tuft's Assessment of Motor Performance (TAMP) (Gans et al., 1988)	• Rehabilitation—stroke, brain injury	• Comprehensive motor assessment for use with adults, with 32 mobility, ADL and communication test items rated on a six-point proficiency scale and time recorded for task completion
Acute care index of function (ACIF) (Van Dillen and Roach, 1988)	• Patients in acute care hospitals	• Measures items in categories of mental status, bed mobility, transfers and mobility (wheelchair and ambulation)
Motor Assessment Scale (MAS) (Carr and Sheperd, 1998)	• Stroke	• Evaluates performance of 7 functionally-based tasks • Performance rating is based on movement patterns used to accomplish task
Emory Functional Ambulation Profile (EFAP) (Wolf et al., 1999)	• General rehabilitation	• Assesses performance of walking ability based on varying environmental contexts
Peabody Gross Motor Scales (Folio and Fewell, 2000)	• Pediatrics (birth-6 yrs)	• Evaluates general gross motor skills, including crawling, walking, changing positions, ball throwing and jumping
Timed up and go test (Podsiadlo and Richardson, 1991)	• Geriatric, rehabilitation, falls risk assessment	• Measures time to complete task: stand up from a chair, walk 10 ft, turn around, walk back, sit down
Functional Reach Test (Duncan et al., 1990)	• Geriatric, rehabilitation, falls risk assessment	• Tests reaching ability, measures how far patient can reach forward from a standing position

*Refer to references listed to determine each measure's proper use and measurement properties.

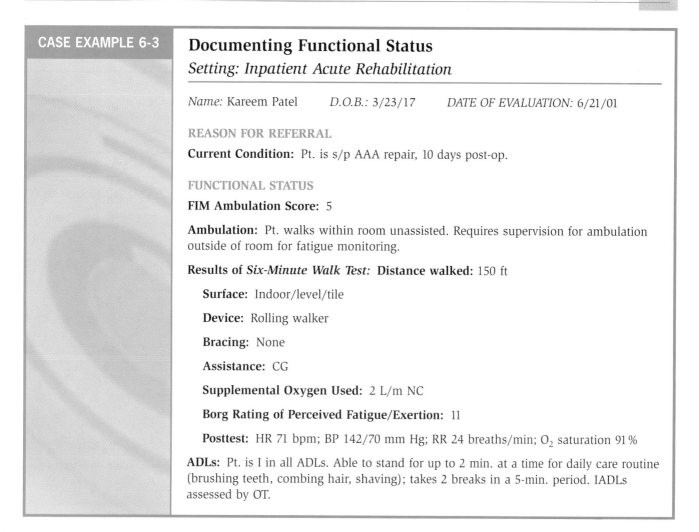

CASE EXAMPLE 6-3

Documenting Functional Status
Setting: Inpatient Acute Rehabilitation

Name: Kareem Patel   *D.O.B.:* 3/23/17   *DATE OF EVALUATION:* 6/21/01

REASON FOR REFERRAL
Current Condition: Pt. is s/p AAA repair, 10 days post-op.

FUNCTIONAL STATUS
FIM Ambulation Score: 5

Ambulation: Pt. walks within room unassisted. Requires supervision for ambulation outside of room for fatigue monitoring.

Results of *Six-Minute Walk Test:* Distance walked: 150 ft

   Surface: Indoor/level/tile

   Device: Rolling walker

   Bracing: None

   Assistance: CG

   Supplemental Oxygen Used: 2 L/m NC

   Borg Rating of Perceived Fatigue/Exertion: 11

   Posttest: HR 71 bpm; BP 142/70 mm Hg; RR 24 breaths/min; O_2 saturation 91%

ADLs: Pt. is I in all ADLs. Able to stand for up to 2 min. at a time for daily care routine (brushing teeth, combing hair, shaving); takes 2 breaks in a 5-min. period. IADLs assessed by OT.

SUMMARY

- Functional status is likely the most important component of physical therapy documentation and is used to justify the need for physical therapy services.

- For an activity to be considered functional in nature, it must (1) be meaningful to an individual and (2) help an individual to fulfill his or her roles.

- A specific function cannot be separated from the context in which it was performed. Thus context-specific documentation is a critical feature of reporting a patient or client's functional status.

- Rather than document all possible functions, the PT should prioritize the functions that are most meaningful to the patient and are amenable to change.

- Therapists must document specific functional problems that are related to certain impairments or a pathologic condition. In preventative care this may include documenting *potential* disability, functional limitations, or both.

- Skill can be defined as the ability to achieve a desired outcome with *consistency, flexibility,* and *efficiency.* These components can be used to provide reliable and measurable documentation of functional status, beyond level of assistance.

EXERCISE 6-1

Identify the errors in the following statements documenting Functional Status. Errors could include: not enough detail, not measurable, context not specified, or negative connotation or labeling. Indicate the specific word or words that are problematic, if applicable. Rewrite a more appropriate statement in the space provided.

Statement	What is Wrong?	Rewrite Statement
Example: Demonstrates poor sitting balance.	Not measurable; "poor" is vague terminology; better to describe sitting ability in a specific context.	Pt. is able to sit for 10 seconds on side of bed, feet flat on floor, before losing balance to the right side. Needs assistance to return to an upright sitting position.
1. Able to walk 50 ft.		
2. Able to eat with a spoon with occasional assistance.		
3. Pt. is confined to using a wheelchair for long-distance mobility.		
4. Able to climb a few stairs.		
5. Can throw a ball but cannot catch one.		
6. Can walk on uneven surfaces.		
7. Pt. is not motivated to walk.		
8. Dresses upper body with difficulty.		

Statement	What is Wrong?	Rewrite Statement
9. Walks slowly.		
10. Pt. doesn't drive.		
11. C/o pain during standing.		
12. Transfers with assistance.		
13. Pt. can lift various size boxes.		
14. Pt. can't get up from a low chair.		
15. Pt. is having trouble sitting for extended periods at work.		

EXERCISE 6-2

The following statements are taken from various sections of an initial evaluation report written in a hospital setting. Extract the information that is appropriate to include in the Functional Status section of the report. Rewrite this information in the space provided below, organizing the information into subheadings based on the areas of function that are being documented (e.g., ambulation, bed mobility, transfers, etc).

1. Pt. will return to work in 4 wks.

2. Pt. is s/p CABG × 4.

3. Pt. walks 200 ft. in hospital hallway c̄ supervision, c̄ ↑ in HR to 120 bpm.

4. Pt. performs daily morning routine of brushing teeth and shaving in 5 min s̄ SOB while standing.

5. Pt. can ↑↓ 10 stairs with 1 railing, step over step, in 22 sec.

6. Strength B knee extension 4/5.

7. Pt. has 20 yr. history of IDDM.

8. Pt. transfers from bed to W/C c̄ supervision.

9. B ankle pitting edema c̄ circumferential measurement L > R by 0.75″.

10. PROM B LE WFL x̄ B ankle DF to 0°.

11. Pt. can ↑↓ 6″ and 8″ curbs c̄ CG.

12. Pt. performed ADLs I before surgery.

13. Able to dress upper body I'ly; requires mod A to reach down to put on pants and don shoes and socks from a seated position.

FUNCTIONAL DOCUMENTATION:

_____

_____

_____

_____

_____

_____

_____

_____

_____

_____

_____

_____

_____

_____

_____

EXERCISE 6-3

For each of the occupations listed below, write a list of functional activities that would be most appropriate to document in the Functional Status section for a theoretical patient. They should be functional activities specific to the patient's particular life role.

Bus driver

_____

_____

Homemaker

_____

_____

College student

_____

_____

Administrative assistant

_____

_____

Professional basketball player

_____

_____

CHAPTER 7

Documenting Impairments

LEARNING OBJECTIVES

After reading this chapter and completing the exercises, the reader will be able to:

1. Define impairments.
2. Describe the categories in the *Guide's* tests and measures that relate to impairments.
3. Document impairments concisely using appropriate terminology and abbreviations.

DEFINING AND CATEGORIZING IMPAIRMENTS

According to the Nagi model, impairment is defined as "anatomical, physiological, mental, or emotional abnormalities or loss" (Jette, 1994). PTs evaluate a wide range of impairments. The impairments that a therapist chooses to evaluate for a particular patient are based on the patient's functional limitations and his or her underlying pathologic condition. A comprehensive consideration of impairment assessment is beyond the scope of this chapter. (See O'Sullivan & Schmitz, 2001, for more information on impairment assessment.)

The *Guide to Physical Therapist Practice* provides a list of the tests and measures commonly used by PTs. Of the 24 groupings in Chapter 2 of the *Guide,* 18 include some components of impairment-based tests and measures (Figure 7-1). As emphasized in Chapter 6, the *Guide* does not organize tests and measures according to impairment and function. This differentiation is often difficult and may be perceived as a continuum rather than a strict separation (see Figure 6-1).

When categorizing impairments, it can be useful to create headings that organize Impairment documentation in an evaluation report or progress note. The *Guide* presents a categorization of the tests and measures used in physical therapy. However, impairments many be categorized in many ways depending on the type of medical condition, the facility, and the personal preferences of the therapist (see Case Examples 7-1, 7-2, and 7-3).

CHOICE OF IMPAIRMENTS FOR DOCUMENTATION

As mentioned in previous chapters, the PT need not document the results of every test or measure that has been performed, especially if the findings were negative (i.e., normal). For example, the initial evaluation need not list in an exhaustive fashion the range of motion of every joint and strength of every muscle group. On the contrary, *the impairments section of the note should highlight those impairments that contribute to the observed functional problems or may potentially lead to later disability.* Too much data in the Impairment section can easily obscure the important findings. Checklists or forms that document a large amount of data can be appended to the note to simplify it and not clutter the text with extraneous findings. This strategy is useful for measures such as range of motion (ROM) or manual muscle tests (MMT), which typically are performed throughout the body. In such cases, pertinent findings should be highlighted in the initial evaluation note, while referring the reader to additional documentation.

The general approach of this text is to recommend reporting those results that are relevant to the patient's current condition, and that are necessary to develop an adequate rationale for the diagnosis and intervention plan. (This is sometimes referred to as *documentation by exception.*) Some therapists, however, contend that it is necessary to document the *absence* of impairment so that if an impairment is found later, it is clear when

IMPAIRMENT-BASED TESTS AND MEASURES

- Aerobic capacity/endurance
- Anthropometric characteristics
- Arousal, attention, and cognition
- Circulation (arterial, venous, lymphatic)
- Cranial and peripheral nerve integrity
- Ergonomics and body mechanics
- Gait, locomotion, and balance
- Integumentary integrity
- Joint integrity and mobility
- Motor function (motor control and motor learning)
- Muscle performance (including strength, power, and endurance)
- Neuromotor development and sensory integrity
- Pain
- Posture
- Range of motion
- Reflex integrity
- Sensory integrity
- Ventilation and respiration/gas exchange

FIGURE 7-1

Impairment-based tests and measures.
(From the *Guide to Physical Therapist Practice*, 2001.)

it developed. Although such an approach is usually unnecessary, there are instances when it is appropriate. If a patient is *at risk* for developing an impairment because of the particular medical condition, the absence of impairment should be documented. For example, in a patient with severe diabetes and associated peripheral vascular disease, skin condition of the toes should be checked regularly and documented because tissue necrosis is a genuine risk in these patients.

Documentation of normal findings also occurs when the findings are directly relevant to confirming, refuting, or reshaping the medical diagnosis. For example, if a patient has pain in his or her shoulder and strength and ROM of the neck and shoulder were normal, these specific findings would be very important to document. Therapists often use two general terms, *WNL* (within normal limits) or *WFL* (within functional limits), as a way to indicate "normal" or "typical" findings. Keep in mind, however, that there are no accepted definitions for these terms, and different professionals reading a note may interpret them in different ways. In general, the terms should be avoided except when used to describe the results of a quick screening examination.

Use of tables or pre-printed forms are often helpful during documentation of similar kinds of impairments. Range of motion and manual muscle testing are amenable to use of tables or pre-printed forms for documentation. This enables greater readability and better organization, particularly if a large number of values are being reported (Case Example 7-1). Appendix D provides examples of forms that can be used as a supplement to a standard evaluation for range of motion evaluation. If such forms are used, no line should be left blank. This way the evaluation cannot be doctored by another party without the therapist's knowledge. Also, if a line is left blank, the reason it was left blank is unknown to the reader. The therapist must write one of the following on the line:

1. The results of the test, examination findings, or clinical opinion.
2. *N/T* (not tested) indicates that this item was not tested. This entry in the note should be followed

DOCUMENTING PAIN

Pain is probably the single most common impairment that a PT encounters in clinical practice, and it is not enough to write merely that "Pt. c/o pain in L shoulder," or some similar statement. Instead, the pain symptoms should be documented precisely and completely. Bickley and Hoekelman (1999) have nicely outlined the seven characteristics of a symptom that need to be clarified. Based on their formulation, the essential characteristics of pain that should be documented are:

1. *Location:* Where is the pain? Does it radiate? Is there a discrete locus, or an indefinite area? Use precise anatomic terminology or include a drawing of the precise locus and extent. Many clinics have forms with outlines of the body (anterior and posterior) that can be used to mark the location of the pain. It is best if the patient marks this directly on a form (see Appendix D)

2. *Quality:* What does it feel like? The nature of the pain sensation can vary widely. For example, it may be sharp, burning, stabbing, aching, or throbbing, to name just a few descriptors. It is best to ask the patient to describe the pain and to use the patient's own words in the documentation.

3. *Severity:* How bad is it? The intensity of the pain sensation is often assessed verbally by using a numeric scale (usually 0–10 where 10 is the "worst possible pain) or a visual analog scale (see an example in Appendix D). The severity is then documented as n/10 in the case of the numeric scale or as a % of max in the case of the visual analog scale.

4. *Timing:* When did the pain start? When and how often does it occur? Is it getting better or worse with time?

5. *Factors that make it better or worse:* How is the pain affected by different movements or activities or rest?

6. *Setting in which pain occurs:* Are there environments, personal activities, emotional situations, or other circumstances that bring about the pain?

7. *Associated manifestations:* Are there other symptoms that occur in conjunction with the pain.

EXAMPLE: Pt. reports sharp, stabbing pain in right knee (localized to discrete point in center of patella) during stance phase of walking (3/10 at comfortable walking speed). Pain increases as walking speed increases, is most intense (8/10) during running, and is absent at rest. Onset of pain "about 3 months ago." Pain is gradually worsening, and is now preventing her from exercising or engaging in recreational sports (e.g., tennis).

For documentation of an initial evaluation, the first five characteristics listed above should almost always be included. However, it may sometimes be the case that not all of these characteristics require documentation. For example, *settings* and *associated manifestations* may be unremarkable in a specific case, and therefore do not need to be included in the documentation. When documenting a progress report or daily note, it would be redundant for the therapist to document each of these characteristics, particularly if they had not changed. In a daily note, a therapist may choose to document only the patient's pain rating on the VAS, if all other aspects remain the same.

by a reason the item was not tested or a plan for testing in the future (e.g., "N/T 2° to time constraints—to be evaluated 11/1").

3. *N/A* (not applicable) indicates that this test was not applicable for this particular patient, given his or her diagnosis or condition. The therapist should state why the test/measure is not applicable (e.g., "N/A—pt. is currently on ventilator and unable to get out of bed").

Quantifiable and objective data should be provided for impairment measures or abnormal findings to be useful for diagnostic or evaluative purposes. Therapists should take care to document impairments with clarity and precision, avoiding vague and ambiguous terminology. Terms such as *minimal, moderate, maximal* or *good, fair, poor* are not particularly useful in descriptions of impairments and should be used sparingly in favor of more measurable, quantifiable assessments.

In addition to performing tests and measures directly relevant to the current condition, therapists should perform a *systems review.* This review often includes a limited examination of impairments related to various body systems: cardiovascular/pulmonary, communication ability, integumentary, musculoskeletal, and neuromuscular. For example, for an elderly patient who is referred with shoulder pain, the following information could be documented: blood pressure and heart rate (cardiovascular), language or cognitive deficits (communication ability), skin assessment (integumentary), ROM and strength in LEs in addition to UEs (musculoskeletal), and any neurologic signs such as sensory changes or reflexes (neuromuscular). This would also include, if pertinent, emotional/behavioral responses and learning preferences or special needs. These tests and measures could be separately categorized in a section titled "Systems Review" (see Case Example 7-1), or could be documented along with other impairments (Case Example 7-2).

IMPAIRMENT TESTS AND MEASURES

Many impairment-based measures used in physical therapy are quantitative in nature. Therapists should

CASE EXAMPLE 7-1

Documenting Impairments

Setting: Outpatient

Name: Jose Rodriguez   *D.O.B.:* 12/29/79   *DATE OF EVALUATION:* 2/25/02

Current Condition: Pt. is a 22-year-old male college student c̄ medical diagnosis of R partial ACL tear 2/22/02.

IMPAIRMENTS

Measure	Left Knee	Right Knee
ROM		
Knee extension	0-10°	–5
Knee flexion	0-145°	5-120°
STRENGTH		
Knee extension	5/5	4/5
Knee flexion	5/5	4/5
REFLEXES		
Patellar tendon	2+	2+
Achilles tendon	2+	2+
SPECIAL TESTS	–Lachman	+Lachman
	–Pivot shift	+Pivot shift
	–McMurray	+McMurray for medial and lateral menisci
CIRCUMFERENTIAL MEASUREMENTS		
Inferior pole of patella	34.0 cm	35.0 cm
Superior pole of patella	35.0 cm	36.0 cm
3 cm proximal to superior pole of patella	36.5 cm	37.5 cm
15 cm proximal to superior pole of patella	43.0 cm	42.5 cm

Palpation: Moderate calor and tenderness along the anteromedial joint line, as well as MCL and medial meniscus.

Pain: Pain 3/10 on VAS at rest; throbbing, aching pain mid-patellar region. 7/10 on VAS while ↑↓ stairs and doing any twisting motion; described as jabbing pain mid-patellar region.

Systems Review: UE and LE strength and ROM WNL (with above-noted exceptions). Skin intact. No evidence of cardiovascular problems; HR 60; BP 120/78. Cognition and communication intact.

carefully choose impairment-based measures that have established reliability and validity. Examples of commonly used standardized tests and measures are listed in Table 7-1. A more detailed listing can be found in other references (*Guide to Physical Therapist Practice, Part III;* Cole, 1995; Lewis and McNerney, 1994; Lewis and McNerney, 1997).

ROM assessment and muscle strength testing are two of the most commonly utilized impairment measures for PTs. Both provide numeric data, in number of degrees and strength grade, respectively. While ROM measurements have been generally found to be reliable (Mayerson and Milano, 1987), manual muscle testing has more limited reliability (Frese et al., 1987; Escolar et al., 2001).

Despite this, manual muscle testing continues to be the most commonly used method by physical therapists to measure strength. Other measures, such as hand-held dynamometers, or isokinetic measurements (e.g., peak torque or torque curves) can provide more reliable and quantitative data to evaluate muscle strength and measure its change over time.

Functional strength tests, such as the functional jump test, can provide useful information related to muscle strength (Davies, Wilk, Ellenbecker, 1997). (See Malone, McPoil, Nitz (1996) for more information on strength measures and documentation.) In certain cases, a description of functional strength or motor control is most appropriate (see Case Examples 7-2 and 7-3).

CASE EXAMPLE 7-2

Documenting Impairments
Setting: Nursing Home

Name: Marjorie Jones   *D.O.B.:* 5/12/17   *DATE OF EVALUATION:* 7/3/99

Current Condition: Pt. is an 82 y.o. female who has a diagnosis of Parkinson's disease c̄ history of multiple falls.

IMPAIRMENTS

Vital Signs: HR 68 bpm; RR 15 breaths/min; BP 120/78 mm Hg

Skin Assessment: +2 Pitting edema noted in both lower legs and feet

Posture: Forward head, thoracic kyphosis, posterior pelvic tilt, and flexion at B hips and knees in standing

ROM: Limited PROM as follows: B hip extension -10°; B hip flexion 10-100°; -10° B knee extension -10°; R shoulder flexion 0-160°, ER 0-45°, abduction 0-140°; L shoulder flexion 0-140°, ER 0-40°, abduction 0-120°

Muscle Tone: Moderate rigidity evident in PROM × 4 extremities, all directions.

Motor Control: Able to move all 4 extremities against minimal resistance. Rapid alternating movements of UEs are slowed. Resting tremor B hands; does not interfere c̄ hand fx.

Sensation: Intact to light touch B UEs and LEs.

Balance: *Sitting:* Can reach 6 in outside arm's length to front and both sides; tolerates moderate perturbations with I recovery in all directions. *Standing:* Can reach only 2 in outside arm's length to front and sides; able to tolerate perturbations to balance against minimal force. Stepping strategy used 4/6 trials to backward perturbation; no response 2/6 trials (caught by examiner)

Gait/Ambulation: Pt. walks without an assistive device for short distances on floor (approximately 100 ft to go to nurses' station or recreation room). Pt. exhibits a shuffling gait with foot flat initial contact. She takes small steps and has a fast cadence (140 steps/min). She also has a narrow step width c̄ R foot occasionally crossing midline. Pt. demonstrates occasional freezing episodes while ambulating in room. Hips and knees are flexed, and there is no visible trunk rotation and only slight arm swing.

TABLE 7-1 STANDARDIZED ASSESSMENTS OF IMPAIRMENTS		
	Population	**Purpose**
Fugl-Meyer (Fugl-Meyer et al., 1975)	• Stroke	• Based to a large extent on Brunnstrom's description of the stages of stroke recovery; most items scored on a 3 point scale (0, 1, 2); includes motor function, sensation, ROM, and pain
NIH Stroke Scale (Goldstein et al., 1989)	• Stroke	• Measures neurologic impairments in patients post-stroke
Mini-Mental State Examinations (MMSE) (Folstein et al., 1975)	• Any individual with cognitive deficits, dementia	• Assesses several categories related to cognition, including memory, recall and language (0-30 points)
Berg Balance Scale (Berg et al., 1992)	• Any neurologic condition, elderly, individuals with balance problems	• Measures balance ability on 4-point scale for 14 balance items, such as standing with eyes closed and turning in place
Glascow Coma Scale (Jennett and Teasdale, 1977)	• Brain injury	• Rates of alertness and cognitive awareness in 3 categories (total score range 3-15)
Modified Ashworth Scale (MAS) (Bohannon and Smith, 1987)	• Any neurologic condition (e.g., stroke, brain injury, spinal cord injury)	• Evaluates muscle tone and stiffness on a 5-point rating scale
Rate of Perception Exertion (RPE) (Borg and Linderholm, 1970)	• Cardiopulmonary rehabilitation	• Patients rate their perceived exertion on a 15-point scale (6-20)

Reporting joint range of motion, most commonly in number of degrees, can be susceptible to certain ambiguities. For example, consider the following statement:

Knee extension-flexion ROM is 10°-150°

While the end of flexion range in this statement is clear (150°), the end of extension rage is ambiguous. Does this statement mean that the individual cannot fully extend the knee (10° knee flexion contracture), or does it mean that the individual has 10° of extension beyond the neutral?

The ambiguity arises in trying to report flexion-extension as a single range of values. Although there are accepted ways to do this (see Reese and Bandy, 2002, for an excellent discussion of the different methods of recording ROM values), the best way to avoid ambiguity is to separate the range into two separate components, one for each direction of movement. For example:

Knee flex: 0°-150°
Knee ext: 0°-10°

The unambiguously state that the individual ha 150° of flexion range and 10° of extension beyond neutral. If, instead, the individual has a 10° knee flexion contracture, it would be reported in this way:

Knee flex: 10°-150°
Knee ext: -10°

Note that ROM is always stated as a range of values (e.g., 0°-150°), except in the case where the individual cannot reach the neutral value, in which case the range is stated as a single negative value.

The first rule of reporting ROM values is to be absolutely clear. If necessary, make a detailed and explicit statement of the range. For example:

Right knee has passive flexion range to 150°, but the knee cannot be fully extended to neutral, stopping at 10° of flexion.

This is wordier than the simple statement above, but at least it is unlikely to be misinterpreted.

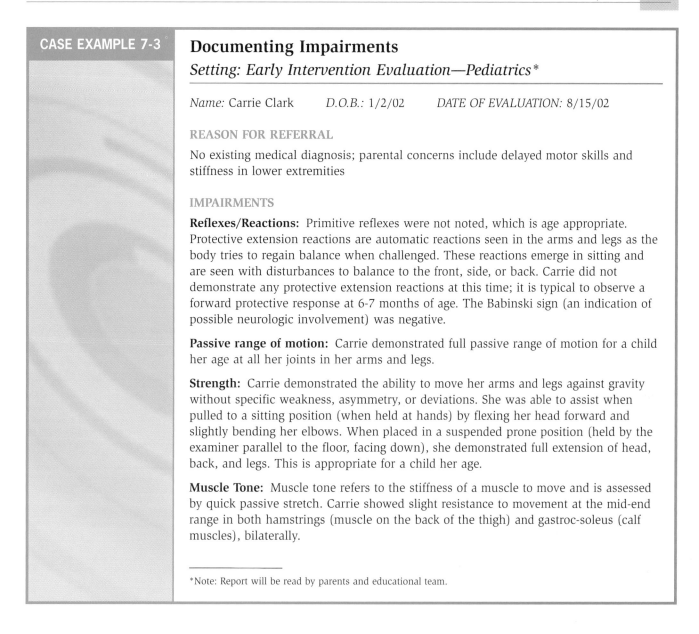

CASE EXAMPLE 7-3

Documenting Impairments

Setting: Early Intervention Evaluation—Pediatrics *

Name: Carrie Clark   *D.O.B.:* 1/2/02   *DATE OF EVALUATION:* 8/15/02

REASON FOR REFERRAL

No existing medical diagnosis; parental concerns include delayed motor skills and stiffness in lower extremities

IMPAIRMENTS

Reflexes/Reactions: Primitive reflexes were not noted, which is age appropriate. Protective extension reactions are automatic reactions seen in the arms and legs as the body tries to regain balance when challenged. These reactions emerge in sitting and are seen with disturbances to balance to the front, side, or back. Carrie did not demonstrate any protective extension reactions at this time; it is typical to observe a forward protective response at 6-7 months of age. The Babinski sign (an indication of possible neurologic involvement) was negative.

Passive range of motion: Carrie demonstrated full passive range of motion for a child her age at all her joints in her arms and legs.

Strength: Carrie demonstrated the ability to move her arms and legs against gravity without specific weakness, asymmetry, or deviations. She was able to assist when pulled to a sitting position (when held at hands) by flexing her head forward and slightly bending her elbows. When placed in a suspended prone position (held by the examiner parallel to the floor, facing down), she demonstrated full extension of head, back, and legs. This is appropriate for a child her age.

Muscle Tone: Muscle tone refers to the stiffness of a muscle to move and is assessed by quick passive stretch. Carrie showed slight resistance to movement at the mid-end range in both hamstrings (muscle on the back of the thigh) and gastroc-soleus (calf muscles), bilaterally.

---

*Note: Report will be read by parents and educational team.

A second problem that sometimes arises with reporting of ROM, especially with students, is confusion between active and passive. Whether the term "range of motion" or "ROM" is used without a modifier, it implies *passive* ROM. If the writer of the note means active ROM, then the word "active" must be stated.

SUMMARY

- Impairment-based documentation should be categorized into test and measure headings.

- Impairment documentation should be selective; it should highlight impairments that contribute to the observed functional problems or may potentially lead to later disability.

- Therapists should consolidate and solidify documentation to include only information that is pertinent for diagnostic or evaluative purposes. This may include documentation of normal findings when appropriate and a Systems Review.

- Whenever possible, impairment documentation should be quantitative. Standardized tests and measures can provide a reliable means for reporting impairments quantitatively.

EXERCISE 7-1

The following statements could be written in an Impairment section of an evaluation report. In the space provided, classify each of the following statements into the appropriate impairment category. This exercise should be completed with reference to the specific tests and measures listed and defined in Chapter 2 of the *Guide to Physical Therapist Practice*.

Impairment Statement	Impairment Category
1. R elbow flexion PROM 0-60°.	_____
2. Walks with uneven step lengths and ↑ weight-bearing time on the R side.	_____
3. Sensation intact B LEs below knee, 10/10 correct responses.	_____
4. Mini-Mental State Examination score 19/30.	_____
5. AROM B UEs WFL.	_____
6. Right facial nerve intact.	_____
7. Circumference mid-patella L knee: 10″; R knee: 9.25″.	_____
8. Rates pain in low back 5/10 on VAS after sitting for 10 min, pain described as aching/throbbing.	_____
9. Skin intact B LE and trunk.	_____
10. Berg balance scale score = 31/56 indicating high risk for falls.	_____
11. Demonstrates antalgic gait pattern.	_____
12. B patellar tendon reflexes 2+/5.	_____
13. B lung fields clear to auscultation.	_____
14. Incentive spirometry in sitting $\bar{c}$ maximal volume = 1750 ml.	_____
15. Pt. has forward head and flattened lumbar lordosis.	_____
16. Pt. is alert and oriented to × 2 (person and place).	_____
17. HR ↑'d to 110 beats/min $\bar{p}$ 5 minutes of walking at 1.0 m/sec.	_____
18. Proprioception sensation impaired L ankle 2/8 correct responses.	_____
19. R hand grip strength 15 kg as measured by hand held dynamometer, avg. 3 trials.	_____
20. Eye movements, smooth pursuit and visual fields intact (cranial nerves II, II, IV, and VI).	_____

EXERCISE 7-2

Identify the errors in the following statements documenting impairments. Errors could include not enough detail, not measurable or objective, or not appropriate for this section. Indicate the specific word or words that are problematic, if applicable. Rewrite a more appropriate statement in the space provided.

Statement	What is Wrong?	Rewrite Statement
EXAMPLE: Demonstrates poor standing balance.	Poor is not measurable.	Pt. unable to stand in place >10 sec $\bar{s}$ LOB.
1. Sensation is impaired.		
2. ROM is moderately limited.		
3. Pt. c/o excruciating pain.		
4. Pt. walks with L knee pain.		
5. Pt. has L leg edema.		
6. Pt. demonstrates a significant ↑ in HR $\bar{c}$ stair climbing.		
7. Pt's. reflexes are hyperactive.		
8. Pt. doesn't know what's going on.		
9. Pt. has abnormal gait pattern.		

Continued

Statement	What is Wrong?	Rewrite Statement
10. Pt. has poor endurance.		

EXERCISE 7-3

The following statements are taken from various sections of an initial evaluation report written in a pediatric outpatient setting. Extract the information that would be appropriate to include in the Impairment section of the report. Categorize the statements using appropriate subheadings (see Case Examples). Rewrite this information in the space provided below.

1. 8 y.o. child with diagnosis of spina bifida.

2. Mild L thoracic C-curve scoliosis.

3. Walks on flat tile surface in hallway 100 feet B loftstrand crutches in 1 min.

4. PROM limited R ankle DF -5°.

5. Proprioception impaired B ankles—0/7 correct responses.

6. Strength B LEs: Hip flexion 5/5 B; hip extension 0/5 B; hip adduction 5/5 B; knee extension R 4/5, L 4+/5; knee flexion R 2+/5, L 3-/5; ankle DF R 2/5, L 2+/5; ankle PF R 0/5, L 1/5.

7. Mother will be instructed in home program to improve ankle ROM.

8. Impaired sensation B LE: L4 dermatome 2/5 correct responses on R, 3/5 on L; L5, S1, S2 dermatomes 0/5 correct responses B.

9. Leg length discrepancy 3/4", R > L.

10. Uses W/C for long distance mobility outside home.

11. Vision is intact.

12. Strength in R ankle PF will increase to 3/5.

IMPAIRMENT DOCUMENTATION:

CHAPTER 8

Documenting the Assessment: The Physical Therapy Diagnosis

LEARNING OBJECTIVES

After reading this chapter and completing the exercises, the reader will be able to:

1. Describe the process of physical therapy diagnosis.
2. Describe the characteristics of the Assessment section of an evaluation report.
3. Appropriately document an Assessment including a physical therapy diagnosis.

This chapter presents the Assessment section of the initial evaluation documentation by the PT. The assessment section is a pivotal section of the documentation. It draws on information presented in the previous sections to arrive at a decision regarding the main problems to be addressed by the PT and the probable causes of those problems. The sections of the initial evaluation that follow the Assessment are used to propose goals and a plan for achieving those goals.

The assessment section is the place where the PT presents his or her *diagnosis* of the patient's condition. The notion that PTs make a diagnosis is a relatively new one and may still be considered controversial. Therefore this chapter begins with an explanation of diagnosis and a consideration of the rationale for diagnosis by PTs. Case Examples 8-1, 8-2, and 8-3 provide sample documentation of the Assessment in various clinical settings.

DIAGNOSIS BY PHYSICAL THERAPISTS

The term *diagnosis* refers to both a process and the product of that process. In a general sense, diagnosis as a *process* is an investigation or analysis of the cause or nature of a condition, situation, or problem. Diagnosis as a *product* is a statement or conclusion from such an analysis. Thus an auto mechanic can diagnose what is wrong with a car, or an electronics technician can arrive at a diagnosis as to what is wrong with a computer. In medicine, diagnosis has traditionally referred to the art or act of identifying a disease from its signs and symptoms or the decision reached by that process.

Diagnosis in physical therapy is controversial because some believe that it should be the sole prerogative of physicians. Indeed, physicians have argued that PTs do not have the training to make a correct diagnosis of a patient's condition, nor are they able to order and interpret the myriad of tests available to the modern physician. However, this perspective is based on a strict definition of diagnosis—that it is the act of determining the nature and location of a pathologic condition. If a broader view is used—that diagnosis is the process by which *any* professional, not just a physician, determines the cause of a problem—then the term can be used to describe the process that PTs use to determine the causes of the problems faced by their patients.

One way to resolve this controversy is to say that the term *diagnosis* refers to a process that all PTs engage in: the act of evaluating the physical and subjective findings to make a decision about whether physical therapy will be helpful to a patient and, if so, what kind of therapy the patient should receive. The physical therapy profession has gradually accepted this terminology (Figure 8-1). The American Physical

Should Physical Therapists Diagnose?

Resolutions of APTA House of Delegates Relevant to Diagnosis

Physical therapy is a health profession whose primary purpose is the promotion of optimal health and function through the application of scientific principles to prevent, identify, assess, correct, or alleviate acute or prolonged *movement dysfunction. (APTA HOD, 1983)*

Physical therapists may establish a diagnosis within the scope of their knowledge, experience and expertise. *(APTA HOD, 1984)*

Physical therapists shall establish a diagnosis for each patient. When the patient is referred with a previously established diagnosis, the physical therapist should determine that clinical findings are consistent with that diagnosis...

Prior to making a patient management decision, physical therapists shall utilize the diagnostic process in order to establish a diagnosis for the specific conditions in need of the physical therapist s attention...

In performing the diagnostic process, physical therapists may need to obtain additional information (including diagnostic labels) from other health care professionals. In addition, as the diagnostic process continues, physical therapists may identify findings that should be shared with other health professionals, including referral sources, to ensure optimal patient care. If the diagnostic process reveals findings that are outside the scope of the physical therapist s knowledge, the physical therapist should then refer the patient to an appropriate practitioner. *(APTA HOD, 1995)*

FIGURE 8-1

Resolutions of the American Physical Therapy Association House of Delegates relevant to diagnosis.

Therapy Association's House of Delegates has shifted its position from one that recognizes the right of a PT to make a diagnosis ("may establish" in 1984; APTA HOD, 1984) to one that requires a diagnosis for each patient ("shall establish" in 1995; APTA HOD, 1995).

Use of the term *diagnosis* as a general term to denote the search for a problem's cause implies that although many features of the process are similar in medical diagnosis and physical therapy diagnosis, there is very often a distinction in the focuses of the two processes. As Figure 8-2 illustrates, in medical diagnosis, the primary focus is the relationship between pathology and impairments. Specifically, impairments (signs and symptoms) are analyzed to determine what disease process, or pathologic condition, is present. In physical therapy diagnosis, on the other hand, the relationship between impairments and functional limitations is typically the primary focus of the analysis, and the purpose of the diagnostic process is identification of the cause of the functional limitations in terms that can be addressed by physical therapy intervention.

To assert, however, that medical diagnosis and physical therapy diagnosis are mutually exclusive processes, with no overlap, would be misleading. Indeed, it can be argued that because of the advances of the past two decades in the understanding of the causes and treat-

ments of movement dysfunction, PTs have become the practitioners who have the appropriate training to develop a proper diagnosis of the causes of movement dysfunction. Although in many cases the diagnoses of the physician and PT remain distinct (see Figure 8-2), at times these diagnostic processes overlap. For example, PTs typically perform a general screening (referred to as "systems review" in the *Guide to Physical Therapist Practice,* 2001) to rule out serious pathologic conditions, such as tumors or heart disease, that are not appropriate for physical therapy intervention. This is sometimes referred to within the physical therapy community as *differential diagnosis.* If evidence of such a pathologic condition is found, the PT must refer the patient to an appropriate practitioner for further testing. This requires the therapist to at least consider the possible pathologic conditions, even if he or she will not verify their presence or absence.

Another example of overlap occurs when the PT uses subjective and objective findings to make a determination of the nature and location of a pathologic disorder. This often occurs in musculoskeletal injuries when the physical examination and subjective examination are the best, and often the only, way to determine the type of tissue damage and its location. In these cases the PT often is the professional most likely to be able to make the specific diagnosis. In fact, such patients often come to the PT with a "diagnosis" that does not identify the pathology at all (e.g., "low back pain" or "shoulder tendinitis"). Thus the boundary between medical and physical therapy diagnosis is not absolute. Indeed, as the knowledge and level of education of PTs continues to increase, the areas of diagnostic competence of the PTs will continue to evolve.

To summarize, diagnosis by physical therapists refers to the process of determining the cause of a patient's functional problems. Sometimes the identified cause will be described in terms of impairments, sometimes in terms of the nature and location of a pathological process. Both types of diagnosis are valid and may potentially be included in the assessment section of the initial evaluation.

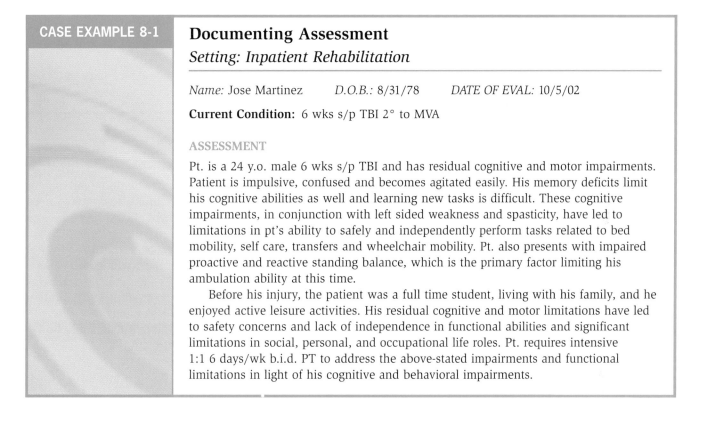

CASE EXAMPLE 8-1

Documenting Assessment
Setting: Inpatient Rehabilitation

Name: Jose Martinez   *D.O.B.:* 8/31/78   *DATE OF EVAL:* 10/5/02

Current Condition: 6 wks s/p TBI 2° to MVA

ASSESSMENT

Pt. is a 24 y.o. male 6 wks s/p TBI and has residual cognitive and motor impairments. Patient is impulsive, confused and becomes agitated easily. His memory deficits limit his cognitive abilities as well and learning new tasks is difficult. These cognitive impairments, in conjunction with left sided weakness and spasticity, have led to limitations in pt's ability to safely and independently perform tasks related to bed mobility, self care, transfers and wheelchair mobility. Pt. also presents with impaired proactive and reactive standing balance, which is the primary factor limiting his ambulation ability at this time.

Before his injury, the patient was a full time student, living with his family, and he enjoyed active leisure activities. His residual cognitive and motor limitations have led to safety concerns and lack of independence in functional abilities and significant limitations in social, personal, and occupational life roles. Pt. requires intensive 1:1 6 days/wk b.i.d. PT to address the above-stated impairments and functional limitations in light of his cognitive and behavioral impairments.

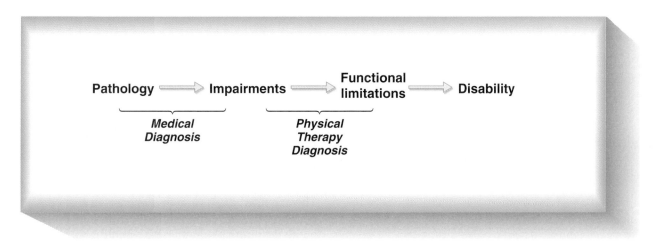

FIGURE 8-2

Medical diagnosis and physical therapy diagnosis involve analysis of the relationships between different levels in the disablement process.

CASE EXAMPLE 8-2	**Documenting Assessment**
	Setting: Inpatient Acute Care

Name: Jesse Goldstein *D.O.B.:* 2/3/40 *DATE OF EVAL:* 5/31/02

Current Condition: s/p Radical hysterectomy 5/29/02 2° to cervical CA

ASSESSMENT

Pt. is a 62-year-old woman s/p radical hysterectomy 2° to cervical CA. Incision site is healing well, but pt. reports significant pain and discomfort in abdominal area. Pt. has limitations in trunk mobility and abdominal strength 2° to surgery. These impairments are limiting pt's independence in bed mobility, transfers, and ambulation, as well as overall comfort in a sitting and supine position. Pt. requires short-duration PT to improve overall strength and endurance, educate regarding appropriate mobility and pain management techniques, and instruct in home program to facilitate recovery.

FORM OF THE PHYSICAL THERAPY DIAGNOSIS

The diagnostic process involves making a clinical judgment based on information obtained from history, signs, symptoms, examination, and tests that the therapist performs or requests. Different methods of diagnosis have been advocated; a few are discussed briefly in Figure 8-3 (see also References). Regardless of the process of arriving at a diagnosis, real questions exist as to the form of the result (the diagnosis). Ideally, the process of diagnosis should involve classifying or labeling the dysfunction. Once the appropriate label has been identified, the intervention would be more or less determined. Physical therapy, however, does not yet have generally agreed on labels or classification systems, although much current research activity is aimed at creating and testing diagnostic systems (Scheets et al., 1999; Delitto and Snyder-Mackler, 1995).

Classification systems should be applied for cases in which they have been shown to be valid. In some cases, involving musculoskeletal disorders, a simple statement of the nature and location of the pathology may suffice for the diagnosis. However, in the absence of agreed on labels, a straightforward descriptive system for documenting the diagnosis is recommended. The system recommended here is based on Guccione's (1991) proposal that a physical therapy diagnosis should express the relationship between impairments and functional limitations. In the preceding chapters, identification and documentation of key impairments that cause or contribute to the critical functional limitations were emphasized. As diagnostic classification systems are tested and validated, these also can be easily integrated into this documentation format.

Examples of physical therapy diagnoses are presented in Table 8-1 to illustrate how a diagnosis might be docu-

mented. For some of the diagnosis examples a medical diagnosis is presented and then two sample PT diagnoses are given, one for an acute condition and one for a chronic condition. The acute-chronic terminology need not be used in actual assessments but is given here to emphasize that the diagnosis may differ depending on the patient's stage of recovery. Note that the physical therapy diagnoses are typically two to three times longer than the medical diagnosis. PTs should be as concise as possible in writing documentation while still capturing the causal relationship in the statement.

The last two examples in Table 8-1 illustrate how a diagnosis regarding the nature and location of the pathology might be stated. Such a diagnosis can be presented simply and succinctly, or it might be written as an extension or elaboration of the medical diagnosis (see Stewart and Abeln, 1993, for further examples of this method). Note that a diagnosis that further defines the nature and location of the pathology is only one part of the diagnostic statement. It is still crucial to determine the causal relationships between impairments and functional limitations (see Figure 8-4).

THE ASSESSMENT SECTION

Organization of the Assessment

The extended discussion of diagnosis in this chapter is necessary because the primary purpose of the Assessment section of the initial evaluation is to present the PT's diagnosis of the patient's problems. In effect the assessment section presents the outcome of the clinical decision-making process. If the first three sections of the initial evaluation have been developed as proposed

Diagnosis – The Process

Inductive methods

- *Inductive reasoning* – the process of deriving general principles from specific facts or instances

- Clinician infers diagnosis from specific signs and symptoms

Hypothetico-deductive methods

- *Deductive reasoning* – a conclusion follows necessarily from stated premises, inferring specific instances from general principles

- *Hypothesis* – a tentative explanation, a conclusion taken to be true for the sake of argument or investigation, an assumption

- Clinician generates hypothesis – *tentative diagnosis*

- Clinician uses deduction to determine the specific signs or symptoms that should be present

- Clinician tests whether deduced signs or symptoms are actually present

Pattern recognition methods

- *Associative memory* — learned knowledge and experience with other patients: a "mental database" of diagnostic labels and associated signs and symptoms

- Clinician matches a specific pattern of signs and symptoms with patterns in associative memory

FIGURE 8-3

Different methods can be used in the process of formulating a diagnosis.

in the preceding chapters, then the assessment should be relatively easy to write. Figure 8-4 reviews the clinical decision-making process and indicates the key elements of the assessment derived from this process.

The items listed in Figure 8-4 are not necessarily documented in the specific order shown. In some cases, especially when the initial evaluation is short and reasonably straightforward, the assessment section might include only the simple statement of the diagnosis. In many cases, however, it is useful to structure the assessment as a summary statement, highlighting the key problems along with the diagnosis and adding a statement of the patient's overall prognosis. One important reason to do this is that some professionals reading the evaluation will skip directly to the assessment. In addition, it is often useful to have a succinct summary statement ready to insert directly for letters to referral sources or insurance companies. It is very important for this reason to minimize use of abbreviations and provide clear, unambiguous statements in this section.

When structured as a summary statement, the Assessment section includes the following components, usually in this order:

1. Summary statement of the patient and the diagnosis.
2. Information clarifying or updating medical diagnosis or pathologic condition.
3. Statement describing patient's functional limitations, key impairments contributing to those limitations, and disabilities or potential disabilities that will result from those limitations.
4. Statement summarizing the patient's potential to benefit from PT and the reasons why PT treatment is or is not indicated.

The Assessment section is the appropriate place to provide specification of the nature and location of the pathologic condition if the PT's examination has revealed this information. The stage of recovery or healing is almost

TABLE 8-1   EXAMPLES OF PHYSICAL THERAPY DIAGNOSES

Medical Diagnosis	PT Diagnosis	Comments
COPD 2° to emphysema with acute pneumonia	*Acute:* Impaired coughing ability resulting in inadequate clearance of airway secretions with potential for fluid accumulation in lungs and infection *Chronic:* Impaired expiratory control resulting in poor endurance during upper extremity functional activities, esp. dressing	Note that in the acute case the primary problem is to prevent secondary complications that might exacerbate the primary pathologic condition. In the chronic case, the problem is functional and the cause is at the impairment level.
s/p medial meniscus tear R knee	*Acute:* Joint effusion, pain, and limitation in range of motion of right knee resulting in potential muscle atrophy and prolongation of healing. *Chronic:* Pain and limitation of range of motion of right knee, knee extensor weakness resulting in difficulty in walking fast and climbing stairs.	The acute case illustrates a common characteristic of orthopedic physical therapy: in the early stages of recovery, the "problem" is often how best to promote healing and prevent secondary complications, or how to return pt. to previous level of activity without harming and allowing repair to heal.
s/p total hip arthroplasty in RLE 2° to osteoarthritis	*Acute:* General weakness; poor transfer and walking skills with immediate risk of complications due to inadequate mobilization. Patient will be ready to function independently at home when independent in transfers and ambulation with walker. *Chronic:* Long-standing limitation in hip range of motion and strength; habitual Trendelenburg-type gait deviation with resulting poor endurance and limited maneuverability in walking	In the acute case, the immediate problem is how to mobilize the patient and to prevent secondary complications. The diagnosis also addresses disability by specifying when patient will be able to function in home.
Low back pain with L4-5 herniated disc	*Acute:* Bilateral hip joint hypomobility is causing hypermobility at L4-5. Pain and muscle spasms are preventing patient from going to work. *Chronic:* Improper postural habits during work activities, hip flexion contracture, and weakness of abdominals have caused decreased support of spine during functional activities, leading to recurrent episodes of pain and inability to work in current job.	In the acute case, the physical therapy diagnosis further specifies or clarifies the medical diagnosis. It also addresses the patient's disability. In the chronic case, the movement dysfunction is producing secondary impairments and exacerbating the pathologic disorder.
L ankle tendinitis	*Diagnosis:* Posterior tibial tendinitis. *Alternate:* Medical diagnosis of L ankle tendinitis is further defined to include posterior tibial tendinitis.	These two examples show how a pathology-level diagnosis might be worded. In each case, the medical diagnosis is nonspecific. Diagnosis may be stated directly or alternatively documented as further defining of the medical diagnosis.
R shoulder pain	*Diagnosis:* R supraspinatus impingement leading to supraspinatus tendinosis. *Alternate:* Medical diagnosis of R shoulder pain is further defined to include supraspinatus impingement leading to supraspinatus tendinosis.	

The Process of Developing a Physical Therapy Diagnosis

1. Disability (or Potential Disability)

- Why has the patient come to, or been referred to physical therapy?
- What is the medical diagnosis?
- What are the patient's desired or required roles, occupations, life goals?
- Does the current condition interfere with these, or does it have the potential to interfere?

> *Identify disability or potential disability . . .*

2. Functional Limitations

- What is the patient's current and prior functional status?
- What are the critical functional activities that the patient needs to perform in order to be able to overcome or prevent disability?

> *Identify functional problems – critical functional activities . . .*

3. Impairments

- Why can't the patient carry out required functional activities?
- What are the causes of the functional limitation?
- What impairments contribute to the functional limitation?

> *Identify causes of the functional problems and contributing factors . . .*

4. Pathology

- Can the medical diagnosis be further specified?
- What is the stage of healing or recovery?
- Is there potential for development of secondary impairments?
- Should the patient be referred to other practitioners?

> *Identify clarifications of medical diagnosis, recovery stage, and requirements for prevention . . .*

FIGURE 8-4

The process of developing a physical therapy diagnosis involves analysis of problems at all levels of the disability model.

always relevant to the overall assessment. Additionally, the PT must always be alert to the possibility of secondary impairments that might develop as a result of the original pathologic disorder. These secondary impairments might in turn exacerbate the pathologic condition or produce new pathologic disorders. It is appropriate to document these risks in the Assessment section.

Examples of Assessment sections are included in this chapter. Keep in mind that these are presented as summary statements; in many instances it is accept-able to leave out the information that has already been presented in other sections of the initial evaluation.

Common Pitfalls in Assessment Documentation

There are several common pitfalls in writing the Assessment section. Usually these result from an overly general or vague statement. For example:

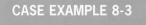

CASE EXAMPLE 8-3

Documenting Assessment
Setting: Health/Wellness Center

Name: Emily Ko   D.O.B.: 9/1/16   *DATE OF EVAL:* 12/2/01

Current Condition: Pt. is 85 y.o. female self-referred for Falls Risk Assessment; hx of 2 falls in past month

ASSESSMENT

Pt. is an 85 y.o. female who is referred for a "falls risk" assessment. Pt. presents with deconditioning, generalized weakness, and poor proactive balance. In addition, pt.'s scores on Berg Balance Scale and Timed Up & Go are indicative of high risk for falls. Pt. is at risk for declining independence and limitations in functional abilities and is at significant risk for falls during dynamic activities such as reaching, walking, or turning. Pt. requires PT intervention to address these specific impairments and functional limitations and to receive education about fall-risk prevention.

Pt has ↓ strength and ROM, which is leading to limitations in ADL.

The problem here is somewhat obvious. This statement could apply to about 90% of all patients seen by a physical therapist. The statements should be more specific:

Weakness in knee and hip extensors and limitation in hip extension PROM prevent patient from being able to perform bed mobility and transfers independently.

Another common example of an overly general statement is the following:

Pt is a good rehab candidate.

This does not sound so bad until we imagine the converse statement:

Pt is a poor rehab candidate.

Neither of these statements is particularly helpful. What do we mean by "good" or "poor"? Both statements merely label the patient, the latter in ways that seem unfair and arbitrary. A better approach is to state more objectively what specific functional limitations might be remediated by a course of rehabilitation therapy. For example:

Pt requires 6-8 sessions of strengthening exercises and functional training in order to become sufficiently skilled in transfers and self-care so that she will be able to function independently at home.

This statement merely implies that the patient is a "good" candidate for rehabilitation because he or she will benefit from it.

If the patient will not likely benefit from further rehabilitation, a clear reason should be given. For example:

Pt has insufficient voluntary movement in fingers of right hand to benefit from therapy to increase usage of right arm.

Or:

Patient is no longer showing improvement in walking velocity and will therefore not benefit from further therapy related to this functional goal.

In general, it is probably not a good idea to make blanket statements about the rehabilitation potential of any patient. Instead, limit statements about prognosis to specific functions for which there is clear evidence one way or the other.

SUMMARY

- The assessment section of the initial evaluation is used to present the physical therapy diagnosis.

- Although the use of the term *diagnosis* by PTs has been controversial in the past, it is now accepted as a legitimate component of physical therapy documentation.

- Physical therapy diagnosis differs from medical diagnosis in its focus. Whereas medical diagnosis uses impairment data to determine the patient's pathologic condition, the focus of the physical therapy diagnosis is on determining the cause of the movement dysfunction, usually by establishing relationships between functional limitations and impairments.

- In addition to the diagnosis, the Assessment section is often structured as a summary statement, restating the medical diagnosis, highlighting key problems, and making a general statement regarding the patient's need for physical therapy.

EXERCISE 8-1

In each of the following cases a therapist's rough notes appear in the left-hand column. Using these as a guide, formulate a plausible Assessment, which includes: a summary statement; clarification of the medical diagnosis (if pertinent); description of relationship between disability, functional limitations, and impairments; and a conclusion statement, summarizing why the pt. requires PT intervention (see Case Examples).

Medical Diagnosis/Pathology	Assessment

CASE 1
59 y.o. man, s/p R THR 2° to osteoarthritis, 3 wks previous. Pt. past acute stage—no significant pain or swelling; incision well healed.

Disability
Sales representative, travels by car, unable to work since surgery.

Functional limitations
Needs assist for transfers into car, walks slowly with walker, up to 100 ft at a time, needs assist on steps.

Impairments
Weakness in R hip flexors, abductors, and extensors; habitual gait deviations from preop antalgic gait.
R hip ✓ and abduction ROM limited.

CASE 2
43 y.o. female with MS diagnosed 3 yrs previous; recovering from recent exacerbation.

Disability
Clerical worker in major downtown office building; rides train and bus to work; resists using cane. Pt. is fearful of falling during commute and needs extra time during commute.

Functional limitations
Requires assist to go up and down steps; walks slowly; walking difficulties exacerbated in crowded places.

Impairments
Only mild weakness; standing balance easily disturbed, esp. when patient is distracted.

Continued

Medical Diagnosis/Pathology   Assessment

CASE 3
39 y.o. female c̄ diagnosis of cervical strain. Onset of
symptoms occurred 6 wks ago.

Disability
CPA at local firm, currently unable to tolerate typical 8-10 hr
work day 2° to symptoms. Majority of time typically spent on
phone and computer.

Functional limitations
Occasionally requires pain medication to assist with sleeping at
night. Unable to talk on phone 2° to pain with phone cradling
position. Unable to tolerate computer work >2 hrs 2° to
increased pain.

Impairments
Static sitting posture presents with a decrease in cervical
lordosis and an increase in thoracic kyphosis. Limited AROM
with R-side flexion and rotation at C-spine. Flexed, rotated,
and sidebent left at C5 and C6. Weakness in bilateral lower
trapezius: 3/5, bilateral middle trapezius/rhomboids: 4/5,
and cervical extensors: 3+/5. Pain rated as 3/10 at rest
and 6/10 after working 2 hrs; described as throbbing and
occasionally shooting.

CHAPTER 9

Documenting Goals

LEARNING OBJECTIVES

After reading this chapter and completing the exercises, the reader will be able to:

1. Describe the important aspects of writing goals at the disability, functional, and impairment levels.
2. Distinguish between short-term and long-term goals.
3. Describe the essential components of a well-written functional goal.
4. Identify poorly written goals and make modifications to goals.
5. Appropriately document disability, functional, and impairment goals for a written report.

This chapter presents the Goals section of the initial evaluation. Establishing anticipated goals and expected outcomes is a critical part of the process of establishing a plan of care for the patient and is one of the cornerstones of physical therapy documentation. The *Guide to Physical Therapist Practice* (2001, p. S38) defines anticipated goals and expected outcomes as

> ... intended results of patient/client management that indicate the changes in impairment, functional limitations and disabilities, and the changes in health, wellness and fitness needs that are expected as the result of implementing the plan of care. (They) also address risk reduction, prevention, impact on societal resources and patient/client satisfaction. The anticipated goals and expected outcomes in the plan should be measurable and time limited.

Physical therapists, in collaboration with patients, set *goals* designed to measure progress toward specific *expected outcomes*. The term *goals* is therefore used in this book to document this process. Through documentation of these goals, therapists express their knowledge of patient's specific problems, formulate the prognosis, and provide the foundation for developing an intervention plan specific to the patient's needs.

Three important aspects about the process of setting expected outcomes should be emphasized. First, in establishing goals, the PT makes a professional judgment about the *prognosis,* that is, the likelihood of functional recovery. The prognosis is, in effect, a prediction about the future, and therefore it depends on a very high level of skill, knowledge, and experience. Nevertheless, it should not be assumed that establishing a prognosis requires years of experience. Indeed, one of the most beneficial aspects of evidence-based practice is the increased availability of information about prognosis.

Second, the process of setting goals is a collaborative effort between the therapist and the patient and often the patient's family and other professionals. Randall and McEwen (2000) have developed this point cogently in an article in *Physical Therapy* entitled "Writing Patient-Centered Functional Goals." They propose a method for writing goals that is very similar to the one proposed in this textbook. The term *patient-centered* is especially useful because it emphasizes that successful therapy mandates that the goals be focused on what the patient wants to accomplish. As they comment, "For goals to be truly patient-centered, they should be relevant to the patient's desired outcomes, not to what the therapist thinks is 'best' for the patient."

Third, goals should guide the therapeutic process throughout its course. If rehabilitation is perceived as a journey, goals are a statement of the destination that the patient and the PT are attempting to reach. For goals to function effectively as a guide they should be referred to during every treatment session, and between sessions as well, as the patient implements his or her "home program." Thus the goals are not simply documented during the initial evaluation; they should be referred to in every daily note or progress note. A method for doing this using the SOAP note format is presented in Chapter 11. Case Examples 9-1, 9-2, and 9-3 provide sample documentation of goals written in initial evaluation reports in various clinical settings.

A TRADITIONAL APPROACH: LONG-TERM AND SHORT-TERM GOALS

The traditional approach to documenting goals has been to distinguish between short-term and long-term goals. Here the distinction is based primarily on the time course of rehabilitation. For example, a typical long-term goal might be:

Patient will walk independently for distances up to 1000 ft outdoors without assistive devices within 1 month.

A short-term goal related to this long-term goal might be

Patient will walk 200 ft on level surfaces indoors using a quad cane and requiring contact guarding within 1 wk.

Thus the concept of a short-term goal is that it is an intermediate step toward achieving the long-term goal. This approach can be useful, especially in rehabilitation settings where treatment may continue for an extended period (Case Example 9-1). However, with changes in

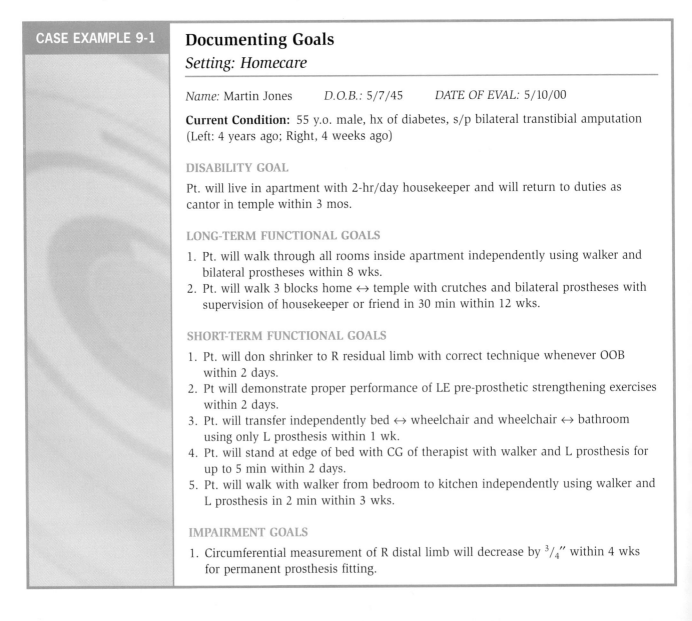

CASE EXAMPLE 9-1	**Documenting Goals**

Setting: Homecare

Name: Martin Jones   *D.O.B.:* 5/7/45   *DATE OF EVAL:* 5/10/00

Current Condition: 55 y.o. male, hx of diabetes, s/p bilateral transtibial amputation (Left: 4 years ago; Right, 4 weeks ago)

DISABILITY GOAL

Pt. will live in apartment with 2-hr/day housekeeper and will return to duties as cantor in temple within 3 mos.

LONG-TERM FUNCTIONAL GOALS

1. Pt. will walk through all rooms inside apartment independently using walker and bilateral prostheses within 8 wks.
2. Pt. will walk 3 blocks home ↔ temple with crutches and bilateral prostheses with supervision of housekeeper or friend in 30 min within 12 wks.

SHORT-TERM FUNCTIONAL GOALS

1. Pt. will don shrinker to R residual limb with correct technique whenever OOB within 2 days.
2. Pt will demonstrate proper performance of LE pre-prosthetic strengthening exercises within 2 days.
3. Pt. will transfer independently bed ↔ wheelchair and wheelchair ↔ bathroom using only L prosthesis within 1 wk.
4. Pt. will stand at edge of bed with CG of therapist with walker and L prosthesis for up to 5 min within 2 days.
5. Pt. will walk with walker from bedroom to kitchen independently using walker and L prosthesis in 2 min within 3 wks.

IMPAIRMENT GOALS

1. Circumferential measurement of R distal limb will decrease by $^3/_4''$ within 4 wks for permanent prosthesis fitting.

the health care system and especially in reimbursement, patients are less likely to be treated over an extended period by a PT. The short-term versus long-term approach to writing goals has therefore become less useful.

WRITING GOALS AT THREE DIFFERENT LEVELS

Although in certain instances establishment of short-term intermediate goals helps to provide a guiding framework for a complex course of rehabilitation, this text advocates a different approach in which the therapist establishes expected outcomes at three different levels: disability goals, functional goals, and impairment goals.

Disability Goals

Disability goals express the expected outcomes in terms of the specific roles that the patient wishes to be able to participate in. These goals provide the "big picture"— what is the overall purpose of the physical therapy intervention? The disability goal for one patient may be to return to work, for another to be able to care for her children, for a third to be able to go to church.

Functional Goals

Functional goals express the expected outcomes in terms of the skills needed to participate in necessary or desired roles. Functional goals are the key component of any goal section and they should never be omitted. For example, a functional goal may be to walk from the bed to the bathroom, to put on a shirt, or to drink from a cup. Because of their importance, functional goals are the focus of much of this chapter.

Impairment Goals

Impairment goals express the expected outcomes in terms of the specific impairments that contribute to the functional limitations. Although the emphasis in this text is clearly on writing functional goals, in some situations one or more goals of therapy involve reduction or elimination of impairments. Therefore in such cases explicit setting of impairment goals is reasonable so that outcomes can be monitored. For example, an impairment goal may be to achieve 4/5 strength in the quadriceps, increase range of motion (ROM) of the knee flexion to 110°, or improve symmetry of step length during gait. Impairment goals also may be viewed as short-term goals

used as benchmarks on the way to attaining functional goals. These goals are particularly important for patients who may have serious limitations in functional abilities, such as immediately after a stroke or spinal cord injury. Changes in impairments, such as strength, may be the only immediate demonstration of improvement in the patient's status, and they may therefore be more sensitive indicators of progress. The goal of therapy is then for the improvements in impairments to ultimately result in improved functional abilities.

LINKING IMPAIRMENT AND FUNCTIONAL GOALS

Impairment goals must always be linked to the functional goals in some way. This linkage should be explicitly stated in the Assessment section. Sometimes therapists link an impairment goal to a functional goal when they are writing the goal. For example, "Pt. will increase ROM R shoulder flexion to 140°, so that patient will be able to reach items in tall cabinet." Rather than taking the time to make this linkage in the Goals section, it is more concise and clear to simply write a functional goal related to reaching items in tall cabinets. The increase in shoulder flexion may or may not be an important impairment/short-term goal, depending on the factors contributing to the functional limitation. A primary reason that such goals often are not useful is that typically more than one impairment contributes to a functional limitation. In the previous example the patient may have a strength deficit in addition to loss of ROM in the shoulder. Thus the patient could attain the goal of improving ROM in the shoulder, but if strength was not improved, the patient would still not be able to reach items in a tall cabinet.

In summary, the focus of therapy should almost always be on achieving critical functional goals, and reaching the impairment goals should be subordinate to attaining the functional goals. Therefore sometimes initial evaluations often will not include explicitly stated impairment goals, but only rarely should the initial evaluation not include explicitly stated functional goals.

FUNDAMENTALS OF WELL-WRITTEN FUNCTIONAL GOALS

Skillful goal writing is deceptively difficult; the PT easily may fall victim to several pitfalls. Therefore the process of learning how to write goals begins by defining the fundamental characteristics of goals and illustrating some of the pitfalls.

CASE EXAMPLE 9-2

Documenting Goals

Setting: Acute Care Hospital

Name: Maria Hispodales   *D.O.B.:* 10/14/35   *DATE OF EVAL:* 11/5/01

Current Condition: 66 y.o. male s/p Right THR 1 day ago 2° degenerative joint disease; PWB R LE.

DISABILITY GOAL

Pt. will return to home to live with his wife, requiring only occasional assistance from daughter and son-in-law for household tasks, within 4 days.

FUNCTIONAL GOALS

1. Pt. will demonstrate proper THR precautions during transfers and dressing 3/3 trials within 1 day.
2. Pt will transfer bed ↔ chair with armrests 3/4 trials within 2 days.
3. Pt. will dress his upper and lower body x̄ socks and shoes with min A from wife within 5 min in 3 days.
4. Pt. will walk independently with walker up to 200 ft in 6 minutes indoors on level carpeted and tiled surfaces within 4 days.
5. Pt. will walk up and down one flight of stairs with single handrail with contact guarding by daughter or son-law within 4 days.

Goals Are Outcomes, Not Processes

The single most important characteristic of goals is that they are outcomes not processes. This is also the characteristic that is most often forgotten, especially by beginning students. A goal is something that the patient, not the PT, will do. The goal defines an end state, not the process that results in that state. The following is an example of a poorly written goal:

Patient will be taught proper precautions following hip replacement surgery.

This is not a goal but a plan for achieving the goal. The goal is for the patient to know the precautions, which can be incorporated into a goal, such as follows:

Patient will be able to state proper hip replacement precautions.

A better, more specific goal would be as follows:

Patient will be able to demonstrate proper hip replacement precautions during bed mobility, sitting, and transfer tasks.

The use of *able to* in these statements is an excellent way to ensure that the goal is defining an end-state, that is, an ability or skill. However, it is not essential in writing the goal. The previous goal could be written without those words as in the following example:

Patient will demonstrate proper hip replacement precautions during bed mobility, sitting, and transfer tasks.

If the patient demonstrates the precautions, it can be assumed that he or she is "able to." Nevertheless, often the PT should at least mentally include the words "able to," especially if the therapist is unsure whether the goal is being properly stated.

Goals Should Be Concrete, Not Abstract

One of the most challenging aspects of writing goals is expressing them in concrete terms. The following goal highlights this challenge:

Patient will demonstrate increased control during reaching movements ...

This statement is hopelessly general and abstract. What is meant by "control during reaching movements"? Ideally, goals should be stated in terms of an *action* or functional task that the individual will perform and must include a concretely stated outcome, such as:

Patient will reach to pick up a cup ...

Too often goals are written in such general terms as to be almost useless. For example, the following goals, written in clinical shorthand, are poorly written:

Ind. ambulation
Ind. ADL
Functional strength in UEs

Although these are clear examples of poorly or at least lazily written goals, often times they may be written in an acceptable form but could be further improved by making them even more concrete and patient-specific. This aspect of goal writing is discussed at the end of this chapter.

Well-Written Goals Are Measurable and Testable

The goal should be stated in such a way that the measurement or testing procedure is explicit. The following goal is neither measurable nor testable:

Good sitting balance

One of (many) problems with this goal is that it is unclear how sitting balance will be tested. In particular, use of terms such as *good, fair,* and *poor* is not recommended because these terms usually imply something different for each person. A better way to write the goal is as follows:

Patient will be able to sit unsupported on the edge of a mat table for up to 1 minute ...

Here the goal is stated in such a way that the test is embedded in the goal itself. One of the reasons why goals are so important is that they provide a way of determining whether progress is being made in the therapy. Therefore frequent testing is essential; ideally, patients are tested on each goal during each treatment session.

Goals Are Predictive

Setting goals requires therapists to generate a prediction. The goal states that the patient will be able to accomplish something in the future that he or she cannot accomplish now. The prediction must be feasible and at the same time challenging. The therapist must also set a specific time within which this goal will be reached. As noted earlier, this aspect is especially challenging for student PTs who have little or no previous experience. Two suggestions may help for students dealing with this problem. First, the rehabilitation literature is an excellent starting point for researching typical times required for achieving certain functional outcomes. Second, goals are not "written in stone." As a patient progresses

in a rehabilitation program, it is appropriate for goals to be revised to reflect the patient's current status and projected capabilities.

The predictions that therapists make in setting goals will therefore not be perfectly accurate because individual patients differ from each other and from the average results in clinical studies. In general, it is better to err on the side of being too optimistic, expecting a bit more from the patients than they may be capable of achieving. If the PT is wrong, then the consequence is that patients do not quite make it, but they are (usually) no worse than if more modest goals had been set. If, on the other hand, the PT errs on the side of being too conservative in patients' goals, the consequence may be that patients do not accomplish what they were capable of. This approach does not advocate unrealistic optimism in setting goals but instead reflects a preference to challenge patients.

Goals Are Determined in Collaboration with the Patient and the Patient's Family

Collaboration with the patient and family is the most obvious of the fundamental characteristics of goals and yet is the most consistently violated principle. Too often the therapist develops a set of goals at the time of writing the initial evaluation, but because the patient is not present at the time, the therapist assumes that these are the goals most important to the patient. Even more detrimental to the rehabilitation process is that the patient may not even be told what the goals are, or they are related only in the most general terms. If the goal is for the patient to be able to walk 500 feet in 2 minutes, why not tell him or her? In our experience, when patients are aware of the specific aspects of a goal, they often work on it on their own time.

A FORMULA FOR WRITING GOALS

Goals have a specific structure, and the first step in learning to write goals is to learn to apply this structure in the process. Applying the principles developed in this chapter, a goal has five necessary components: (1) who will accomplish the goal (Actor), (2) the action that the individual will be able to perform (Behavior), (3) the circumstances under which the behavior is carried out (Condition), (4) a quantitative specification of performance (Degree), and (5) the time period within which the goal will be achieved (Expected Time). These components of a goal and examples are explained further in Figure 9-1. This formula is adapted from a scheme originally developed by Kettenbach (1995).

The five components shown in Figure 9-1 are most readily applied to documentation of functional goals. Some of these components are not pertinent when writing disability or impairment goals (see *Writing Disability and Impairment goals* below). Nevertheless, all properly written *functional* goals should include all five components. Thus the following formula can be applied to writing a functional goal:

$$Goal = A + B + C + D + E$$

Using this formula, the following goal might be constructed:

Mr. McCarthy (Actor) *will walk* (Behavior) *on level surfaces with a walker* (Conditions) *and min A* (Degree) *for a distance of 100 ft. in 2 min* (Degree) *within 1 wk* (Expected Time).

This goal can easily be modified by substituting different components as follows:

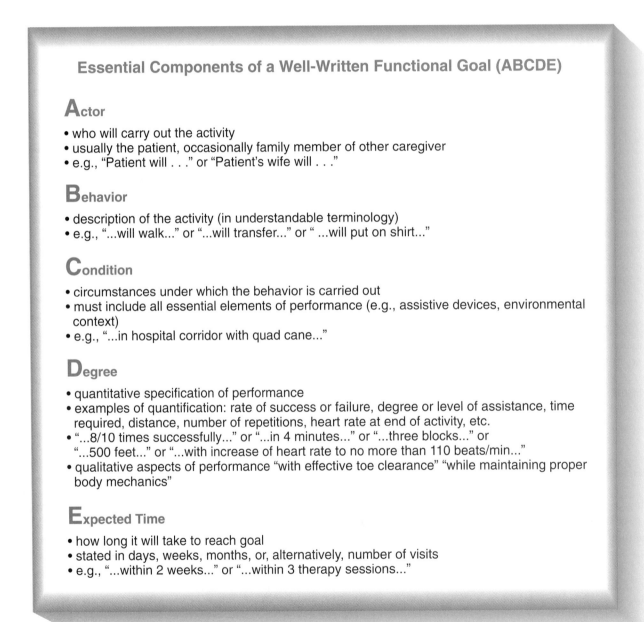

Essential Components of a Well-Written Functional Goal (ABCDE)

Actor

- who will carry out the activity
- usually the patient, occasionally family member of other caregiver
- e.g., "Patient will . . ." or "Patient's wife will . . ."

Behavior

- description of the activity (in understandable terminology)
- e.g., "...will walk..." or "...will transfer..." or " ...will put on shirt..."

Condition

- circumstances under which the behavior is carried out
- must include all essential elements of performance (e.g., assistive devices, environmental context)
- e.g., "...in hospital corridor with quad cane..."

Degree

- quantitative specification of performance
- examples of quantification: rate of success or failure, degree or level of assistance, time required, distance, number of repetitions, heart rate at end of activity, etc.
- "...8/10 times successfully..." or "...in 4 minutes..." or "...three blocks..." or "...500 feet..." or "...with increase of heart rate to no more than 110 beats/min..."
- qualitative aspects of performance "with effective toe clearance" "while maintaining proper body mechanics"

Expected Time

- how long it will take to reach goal
- stated in days, weeks, months, or, alternatively, number of visits
- e.g., "...within 2 weeks..." or "...within 3 therapy sessions..."

FIGURE 9-1

Essential components of a well-written goal (ABCDE).
(Modified from Kettenbach, 1995.)

Mr. McCarthy will walk on level surfaces with a walker and min A for a distance of 500 ft. in 5 minutes (dif- ferent Degree) within 2 wks (different Expected Time).

Or:

Mr. McCarthy will walk outdoors on uneven surfaces with a cane (different Conditions) and min A for a distance of 100 feet in 2 min within 1 wk.

Thus a wide range of goals can be constructed by mixing and matching the different components. The benefits of this approach are twofold. First, goals will be properly written, that is, not missing any essential components. Second, this approach is designed to encourage functionally oriented goals because the focus is on the patient and the action he or she will be performing.

THE ART OF WRITING PATIENT-CENTERED GOALS: GOING BEYOND THE FORMULA

If the writing of good documentation can be said to be an art, then it is in the writing of goals that the artfulness is expressed. The therapist must rise above the formula and create goals, in collaboration with the patient, which will guide the therapeutic process toward the best possible outcome. The key to creating artful goals is to make them "patient-centered." A patient-centered goal is one expressed in terms of specific activities that are meaningful to the patient. The first step is to start with a fairly generic but still acceptable goal:

Mr. McCarthy will walk on level surfaces with a walker and min A for a distance of 100 ft in 2 min within 1 wk.

The goal can be reformulated so that it is more patient-centered as follows:

Mr. McCarthy will walk from his bedroom to his kitchen with a walker and his wife's assistance in 2 min within 1 wk.

A simple change makes the goal much more meaningful to the individual. Another example starts with a fairly generic goal:

Ms. Henry will feed herself independently within 1 wk.

Again, the goal can be reformulated in a way that is more patient-centered:

Ms. Henry will eat a full bowl of dry cereal and milk with a spoon using the right hand in 10 min within 1 wk.

Of course, the assumption here is that Ms. Henry wants to be able to eat cereal in the morning. The patient-centered goal, in addition to being more relevant to the patient, is intrinsically more testable and measurable.

Randall and McEwen (2000) state that the main reason for writing patient-centered functional goals is that "people are likely to make the greatest gains when therapy and the related goals focus on activities that are related to them and that make a difference in their lives." The key to this is taking the time to discuss the goals with the patient so that the goals are formulated in terms that are meaningful to him or her. Then the goal is stated in as concrete a manner as possible.

WRITING DISABILITY AND IMPAIRMENT GOALS

In this discussion of writing goals, most of the discussion has focused on techniques that are appropriate for writing functional goals. Factors that should be considered when the PT writes disability goals and impairment goals are now considered.

Disability Goals

Generally, disability goals can and should be written just as functional goals are written. The difference is that the activity that is the subject of the goal is stated in more general terms than it would be in a functional goal. Disability goals should each have at least four of the five critical components of a well-written functional goal: Actor (A), Behavior (B), Condition (C), and Expected time (E). The Degree (D) may not be necessary when writing disability goals (see Example 3 below). The following statements are examples of disability goals:

Example 1: *Mr. Rasheed (A) will return to work (B) as a bus driver (C) able to accomplish all regular duties (D) within 1 mon (E).*

Example 2: *Ms. Loring (A) will take care (B) of her two children at home (C) without daytime assistance (D) within 2 mons (E).*

Example 3: *Mr. Fox (A) will attend (B) church services (C) within 6 wks (E).*

Example 4: *Ms. Samson (A) will return (B) to jogging for fitness and recreation (C) 4×/wk (D) within 2 mons (E).*

In disability goals, the Condition typically clarifies the nature of the activity or activities. These goals make little sense if they are not followed up by functional goals that detail the specific functional skills needed to fulfill these roles. It may not always be the case that the functional goals will directly lead up to the disability goal. The disability goal may be a goal that is not attainable for several months, which may be beyond the patient's expected duration of treatment in the current setting. This is illustrated in Case Example 9-3. In this case, the patient will likely undergo two separate episodes of PT—one immediately after the accident (for which the goals are listed), which may only last a few weeks, and another episode after the fractures have healed. The disability goal, however, is still stated as a long-term outcome for the patient—to return to school in her full capacity.

Impairment Goals

Impairment goals are considered optional for most evaluation reports. They should be included only if specific impairment-level objectives will be worked on during therapy. In many clinical settings, these are often referred to as *therapy goals* or short-term goals. Impairment goals must be linked to functional goals. The linkage should be clearly stated in the Assessment section of the initial evaluation. An example of an Impairment goal would be as follows:

Passive ROM of L knee flexion (C) will increase (B) to 110° (D) within 3 wks (E).

In this case, the Condition is ROM of left knee flexion, and Degree is measured in joint ROM. Impairment goals are often not written with the actor specified, as it is assumed that the statement is made with relation to the patient. Furthermore, it would not sound incorrect if a goal read "Pt will increase ROM in R knee." It then appears that the *patient* is doing something specific to increase the ROM. Thus impairment goals are often stated without the actor explicitly specified, although the Behavior (B), Condition (C), Degree (D), and Expected Time (E) should be included. Some more examples include:

Example 1: *Strength R shoulder flexion (C) will increase (B) to 4/5 (D) within 3 wks (E).*

Example 2: *Single limb stance on R leg (C) will improve (B) to 10 sec (D) within 2 wks (E).*

CASE EXAMPLE 9-3

Documenting Goals
Setting: Outpatient

Name: Keisha Brown   *D.O.B.:* 1/9/85   *DATE OF EVAL:* 2/12/01

Current Condition: 16 y.o. female s/p fx R distal tibia and fx R proximal humerus 1 wk ago 2° to MVA; NWB R LE.

DISABILITY GOAL

Pt. will attend regular classroom in high school and participate in all activities, including extra-curricular sports, within 4 months.

FUNCTIONAL GOALS

1. Pt. will demonstrate proper performance of home program of active exercises within 3 days.
2. Pt. will transfer wheelchair ↔ car using stand-pilot transfer with min A of father or mother within 2 wks.
3. Pt. will use motorized wheelchair independently in school hallways, elevators, and outside paved areas, while effectively avoiding obstacles and keeping up with peers within 2 wks.

IMPAIRMENT GOAL

1. Pt will tolerate R leg in dependent position for 30 min within 1 wk.

Example 3: *Pain in R shoulder (C) will decrease (B) to 2/10 on VAS (D) within 1 wk (E).*

Example 4: *Circumference of wound (C) will decrease (B) to 2 cm (D) within 4 wks (E.).*

When impairment goals are written, the Assessment section of a report should clearly state that the specific impairments are contributing to the patient's functional problems. For example, if a goal is set to increase shoulder strength, then it should be clearly documented in the Assessment that weakness of shoulder musculature is contributing to the patient's functional limitations.

A common pitfall when documenting impairment goals is to not specify the Degree (D). Some examples include:

↑ *strength R biceps*
↓ *pain in L ankle*

These goals are not well written because they do not include specific measures. In the first example, if a patient's strength increased even a minimal amount, the goal could be met. This might make it difficult to justify the need for continued intervention to achieve even greater strength in the biceps. If, however, the amount of strength (e.g., manual muscle testing grade) was specified as a goal, this would allow all involved parties—patient, therapist, MD, third-party payors—to be aware of the specific expected outcomes.

DETERMINING EXPECTED TIMES FOR GOALS

Determining the appropriate expected time frames for a goal can be particularly challenging. Inevitably, the physical therapist makes an educated guess about how the pathologic condition, medical history, and many other factors will affect how quickly a patient will achieve a goal. While determining expected time frames can be highly subjective, PTs should use current research and their clinical experience and judgment to determine the most reasonable time frame.

Expected time frames are typically written in weeks. In certain settings where the length of stay is typically short, such as acute care hospital settings, goals can be set in terms of days. Time frames can also be written in terms of number of PT sessions by which they are likely to be achieved (e.g. *Pt. will walk 200 ft. in hospital corridor with min A within 6 sessions*).

SUMMARY

- Goals should be distinguished as to whether they are disability goals, functional goals, or impairment goals.

- Well-written goals have certain fundamental characteristics. They are focused on outcomes, not processes. They are concrete, not abstract. They are measurable and testable. They are predictive and are based on collaboration between therapist and patient.

- A functional goal has five essential components: the Actor, the Behavior, the Condition, the Degree, and the Expected Time.

- Although these components can be used to construct a goal in a mechanical way, therapists are expected to go beyond the formula to create goals that are patient centered, that is, stated in terms of activities and environments that are meaningful to the patient.

EXERCISE 9-1

For each goal, indicate what type of goal it is (Disability, Functional, or Impairment). Write one or more letters in the box at the right to indicate the missing or problematic component (A, Actor; B, Behavior; C, Conditions; D, Degree; E, Expected time). More than one component may be missing or problematic in a single example. Rewrite each goal in the space below, adding or changing the missing or problematic components using plausible details. Identify A, B, C, D, and E in each answer.

EXAMPLE: Patient will walk 300 ft in 4 minutes using walker and require contact guarding.

Answer: Patient (A) will walk (B) on level hallway surface (C) 300 ft (D) in 4 min (D), using walker (C) and requiring contact guarding (D) within 5 days (E).

Type: Functional
Problem: C, E

1. Independent in transfers in 2 wks.

   Type:

   Problem:

2. Patient will be functional in ADL within 3 wks.

   Type:

   Problem:

3. Return to work in 3 mon.

   Type:

   Problem:

4. Increased strength in quadriceps to 5/5 bilaterally.

   Type:

   Problem:

5. Pt. will ↑↓ 1 flight of stairs in 1 min.

   Type:

   Problem:

6. Pt. will demonstrate increased R hip ROM.

_____

_____

Type:

Problem:

7. Pt. will return to school.

_____

_____

Type:

Problem:

8. Maintain upright posture while sitting.

_____

_____

Type:

Problem:

9. Pt. will get from his room to therapy.

_____

_____

Type:

Problem:

10. Pt. will perform 10 reps of straight leg raises.

_____

_____

Type:

Problem:

EXERCISE 9-2

Identify the errors in the following statements documenting *Functional Goals*. Errors could include: not a functional goal (disability or impairment), reflects a process (not an outcome), not concrete, context not specified, not measurable, and not predictive. Indicate the specific word or words that are problematic, if applicable. Rewrite a more appropriate statement in the space provided.

Statement	What Is Wrong?	Rewrite Statement
EXAMPLE: Transfers will improve.	Not measurable, context not specified.	Pt. will transfer from bed ↔ w/c c̄ min A, within 1 wk.
1. Patient will experience less pain.		
2. Pt. will progress from a walker to a cane within 3 wks.		
3. Educate patient on hip precautions within 2 sessions.		
4. Return to work.		
5. Pt. will walk with a normal gait pattern within 4 wks.		
6. Pt. will walk independently with a quad cane for distances up to 500 feet within 3 wks.		
7. Pt. will be I in all activities in 2 wks.		
8. Pt. will ascend and descend stairs within 3 days.		
9. Patient will not have pain when reaching.		
10. Strength R knee / will increase to 4/5.		

CHAPTER 10

Documenting the Intervention Plan

After reading this chapter and completing the exercises, the reader will be able to:

1. Identify and describe the components of documentation of an intervention plan.
2. Appropriately document an intervention plan as part of an initial evaluation.
3. Discuss the importance of documenting informed consent.

The Intervention Plan details the physical therapy techniques and procedures that will be utilized to accomplish the stated functional goals. In this section of the report, the PT documents the plan of care to be carried out in future sessions until the goals are reached and records any interventions that may have already been completed during the examination process.

In documenting the intervention plan the PT usually states the proposed frequency and duration of physical therapy visits, in addition to a tentative date for reevaluation. The PT then describes the interventions, preferably prioritizing them in descending order. Categorizing the interventions into the three distinct areas outlined by the *Guide to Physical Therapist Practice* (2001) can help organize this section (Figure 10-1). These three categories are (1) coordination, communication, and documentation; (2) patient-related instruction; and (3) procedural interventions. This categorization is useful because therapists often focus exclusively on describing the procedural interventions and minimize or even omit interventions involving coordination of care, communication with individuals involved in the patient's care, and patient-related instruction. Thus listing each of these three categories helps to ensure that all aspects of physical therapy interventions are addressed.

INTERVENTION CATEGORIES

Coordination/Communication

The therapist should document the coordination of care that occurs directly with a patient, his or her family members, or any individuals directly involved in the patient's care. Such individuals may include PTAs, other medical personnel, caregivers, or teachers:

Diagnosis and plan of care were discussed with PTA, who met pt. and pt.'s family at the completion of the evaluation.

In an initial evaluation report the PT also reports his or her plan for any anticipated coordination or communication that is relevant to physical therapy:

Pt.'s HHA will be instructed in appropriate guarding during standing activities and ambulation to maximize pt.'s safety while facilitating active participation by pt.

(PT will) coordinate with John's SLP re: strategies to maintain upright positioning in W/C, and possible use of adaptive equipment during mealtimes.

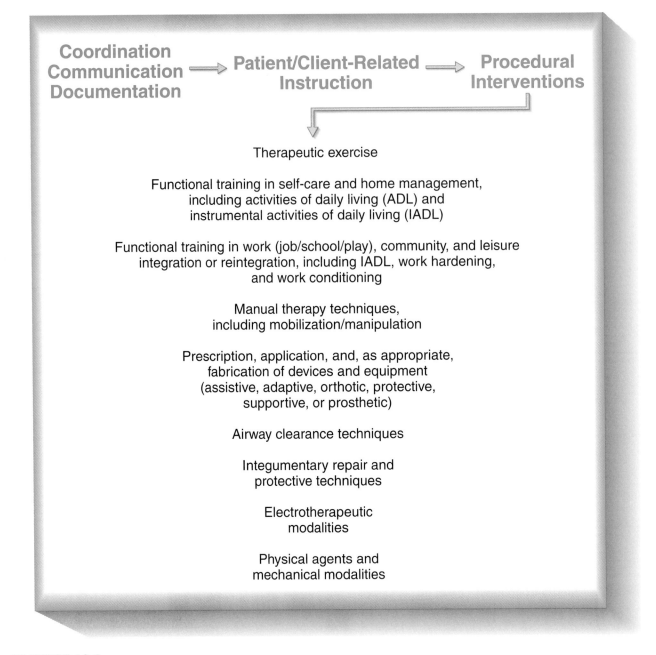

Coordination
Communication ⟹ Patient/Client-Related ⟹ Procedural
Documentation Instruction Interventions

Therapeutic exercise

Functional training in self-care and home management,
including activities of daily living (ADL) and
instrumental activities of daily living (IADL)

Functional training in work (job/school/play), community, and leisure
integration or reintegration, including IADL, work hardening,
and work conditioning

Manual therapy techniques,
including mobilization/manipulation

Prescription, application, and, as appropriate,
fabrication of devices and equipment
(assistive, adaptive, orthotic, protective,
supportive, or prosthetic)

Airway clearance techniques

Integumentary repair and
protective techniques

Electrotherapeutic
modalities

Physical agents and
mechanical modalities

FIGURE 10-1

The three components of physical therapy intervention reprinted with permission from the *Guide to Physical Therapist Practice (2001)*.

Patient-Related Instruction

All physical therapy intervention involves some aspect of patient education or instruction. This section should include a general description of the nature of the instruction. For example, the therapist can report:

Patient will be instructed in care of wound.

Although the specific details of this instruction may not need to be documented in the evaluation report, inclu-sion of any educational materials given to the patient to be kept in the medical record or chart is helpful. Another example that could be included in a report is:

Pt. will be educated on proper positioning in bed.

It could be argued that this statement does not provide enough detail about specifically what is meant by "proper positioning" or why positioning is important for this patient. An alternative documentation might be:

Pt. will be educated on positioning self in side-lying position with pillow between knees to maintain back alignment and improve comfort while sleeping.

Procedural Interventions

The Procedural Interventions section of the Intervention Plan can include a wide range of interventions, from therapeutic exercise to training in self-care skills to airway clearance techniques (see Figure 10-1). First and foremost, documentation of procedural interventions should flow logically and systematically from other aspects of the report. For example, if stair climbing is identified as a functional limitation and improved speed and efficiency in stair climbing is listed as a functional goal, then part of the intervention would logically entail training in stair-climbing skills (see Case Examples 3-1 and 3-2 for complete reports). Sometimes, however, the justification for physical therapy interventions is not so readily apparent. For example, therapists use electrotherapeutic modalities for many different reasons, including muscle reeducation and reduction of swelling. In situations in which the purpose for using a particular intervention is not clear, the therapist must take the time to document in the report a concise rationale for the intervention chosen. For example:

NMES to R quads for muscle re-education.

US to proximal extensor carpi radialis to promote tissue healing.

As with other sections of the physical therapy report, documentation of procedural interventions should be detailed appropriately. For example, simply stating "gait training" is too vague. Specification of more detail about the gait training, such as to improve safety during outdoor ambulation or to improve endurance, speed, or efficiency of gait pattern, is essential. Alternatively, providing too much detail in this section wastes the therapist's time and clouds the report with extraneous information. For example, if progressive resistive strengthening exercises for the right quadriceps and hamstrings is one of the procedural interventions for a particular patient, the PT need not document the specific number of repetitions, sets, positioning, or exact types of exercises that will be performed. Similarly, documentation of modalities in the initial evaluation need not include specific parameters. This information is more appropriately conveyed in each daily note documentation, as the parameters are likely to change over the course of the episode of care.

Interventions listed under procedural interventions include only those that will be carried out by a PT or PTA. The intervention plan should be written in such a

---

CASE EXAMPLE 10-1

Documenting Intervention Plan
Setting: School-Based Pediatrics

Name: Jason Press   *D.O.B.:* 3/15/93   *DATE OF EVAL:* 9/10/01

Current Condition: Duchenne's muscular dystrophy

INTERVENTION PLAN

Jason will be seen for PT 3 days/wk during school year, 30-min sessions; formal reevaluation in 1 yr.

Coordination/Communication: Discuss possibility of B AFOs with home-based PT. Will educate paraprofessional in techniques to assist in transfers.

Patient-Related Instruction: Jason will be instructed in optimal strategies to maximize Jason's independence in performing transfers and during classroom ambulation while monitoring fatigue.

Procedural Interventions:
- Gait training in classroom and in hallway to maximize safety and endurance.
- Active and passive ROM exercises and strengthening exercises for B LEs, specifically quads, hip extensors, and ankle musculature.
- Balance training in standing to address limitations in reactive balance during classroom activities and gym class.
- Stair climbing trng to manage carrying books and maintaining safety.

CASE EXAMPLE 10-2

Documenting Intervention Plan

Setting: Acute care hospital

Name: Joseph Jacobs   *D.O.B.:* 6/17/30   *DATE OF EVAL:* 11/1/00

Current Condition: 1 day s/p right total hip replacement, PWB R LE.

INTERVENTION PLAN

Pt. will receive PT 2 ×/day, 30-min session; anticipated D/C 11/4/00.

Coordination/Communication: F/u with hospital SW re: d/c plan and necessary adaptive equipment—raised toilet seat, tub bench, walker.

Patient-Related Instruction: Pt. instructed in total hip precautions and exercises (hip isometrics, ankle pumps, glut sets, quad sets) pre-operatively on 10/20/99 (handout given). Will continue reviewing precautions and exercises each session. Exercises to be performed 3 ×/day.

Procedural Interventions:
- AROM exercises B LEs—progression from ankle pumps, glut sets, and quad sets to active knee flexion/extension, hip flexion, abduction, and extension following THR precautions.
- Bed mobility and transfer trng while maintaining hip precautions, maximizing independence.
- Balance training in standing to improve standing tolerance during functional activities.
- Gait training for short distances (10-20 ft) with standard walker, progressively increasing distance and ↓ing VCs for safety and foot placement.
- Elevation trng: curbs and stairs to promote independence and safety.

---

way that the reader knows the intervention requires the skill of a PT. For example, stating simply "ambulation" as part of the intervention plan does not suggest skilled intervention. Simply walking with the patient could be performed by nursing staff or by an aide. Instead, the documentation should state "gait training," with emphasis on the specific aspects of gait that are being addressed (e.g., "gait training c̄ manual and verbal cueing to improve foot clearance"). This type of training requires skilled intervention of a PT or PTA.

Therapists should document only those interventions that are within the scope of physical therapy practice. This section should not include reports of interventions performed by other medical professionals. Rather, this information should be described either in the coordination/communication heading or in the Reason for Referral section.

DOCUMENTING INFORMED CONSENT

The principle of informed consent is integral to health care. Whereas traditionally such consent was taken for granted, the modern approach is to verify informed consent in writing. Documenting informed consent has two benefits: it serves as evidence that informed consent was obtained, in case there is a dispute at a later date; and (perhaps more importantly) it serves to remind practitioners to take this crucial last step before beginning treatment.

Documenting informed consent can be done either by having the patient (or responsible family member) sign a standard form, or by reporting that consent was obtained at the end of the written initial evaluation. In the absence of a standard form, an appropriate variant of the following statement should be inserted at the end of the Intervention Plan section:

The findings of this evaluation were discussed with [insert name of patient or responsible party] *and he* [or she] *consented to the above intervention plan.*

If the patient is a minor, or not competent to give informed consent, then the evaluation and intervention plan should be discussed with a responsible person (e.g., parent or spouse). If other persons are present during the discussion of informed consent, indicate who they were.

Finally, the concept of informed consent implies that the patient or responsible party has the right to *not* consent to the recommended intervention plan, either in whole or in part. If that occurs, the PT should indicate in detail what parts of the intervention plan the patient disagrees with and briefly summarize the reasons given.

SUMMARY

- The therapist documents the details of the patient's functional limitations and impairments throughout the functional outcome report; these details should logically lead to specific goals and an appropriate intervention plan designed to achieve those goals.

- The Intervention Plan is typically the last section in a physical therapy report. It reflects the compiling of information from all other aspects of the report and can be the most highly scrutinized section.

- The Intervention Plan includes three types of interventions: coordination/communication, patient-related instructions, and procedural interventions.

- Although the Intervention Plan of an initial evaluation report can be short and concise, it should provide sufficient detail so that the justifications for the chosen interventions are clear.

- Following the Intervention Plan a statement indicating that informed consent was obtained should be included.

CASE EXAMPLE 10-3 | ## Documenting Intervention Plan

Setting: Outpatient

Name: Brian Jones   *D.O.B.:* 9/23/83   *DATE OF EVAL:* 10/15/00

Current Condition: 1 wk s/p R ACL reconstruction

INTERVENTION PLAN

Pt. will be seen for PT 3 days/wk for 4 wks, 45-min sessions. Re-eval in 2 wks.

Coordination/Communication: Consult with athletic trainer at school who will be working with Brian within 2 wks. Follow-up phone call in 5 days with MD to coordinate progression of exercise program.

Patient-Related Instruction: Brian will be instructed in the following:
- PROM exercises for knee flexion and extension for use both in the clinic and at home
- Proper use of CPM machine for passive knee ROM
- Use of ice and elevation to reduce swelling and pain
- Patellofemoral self-mobilization to increase joint mobility
- Isometric quad sets
- Instruction in safe use of crutches in all environments

Procedural Interventions:
- Ultrasound and soft tissue massage to improve circulation and decrease LE edema
- NMES to R quads for muscle re-education
- AROM and progressive resistive strengthening exercises to increase strength of R quadriceps, hamstrings, and gastroc/soleus
- Gait trng to improve safety and endurance during ambulation, including uneven surfaces, ramps, and stairs
- Balance activities in standing to improve RLE stability
- Progressive trng on stationary bike, nordic track, and treadmill to increase cardiovascular and muscular endurance
- Plyometric trng in preparation for return to sport

EXERCISE 10-1

Identify the errors in the following statements documenting the Intervention Plan. Errors could include not enough detail, too much detail; rationale not provided; no indication of skilled services required; or not appropriate for this section.

Indicate the specific word or words that are problematic, if applicable. Rewrite a more appropriate statement in the space provided.

Statement	What is Wrong?	Rewrite Statement
EXAMPLE: Gait training.	Not enough detail. The purpose of the gait trng is not specified.	Gait trng within home with manual and verbal cues to improve gait symmetry and speed.
1. Practice walking.		
2. Apply hot-packs.		
3. Pt. will be able to walk 10 ft to the bathroom.		
4. Pt. will be given strengthening exercises.		
5. Coordinate care with all nursing personnel.		
6. Assess work environment.		
7. Pt. will increase right hamstring strength.		
8. Balance training.		

Statement	What is Wrong?	Rewrite Statement
9. Pt. will receive ultrasound at 1.0 W/cm^2, 1 MHz to R quadriceps (VMO), in a 10 cm area just proximal and slightly medial to right knee, moving ultrasound head slowly in circular fashion for 10 min, each session.		
10. Pt. will take pain relief medication as needed.		
11. Home evaluation.		
12. Reduce R ankle edema.		
13. Teach family to care for patient.		
14. Practice pressure-relief techniques.		
15. E-stim to anterior tibialis.		

EXERCISE 10-2

The following statements are taken from various aspects of an initial evaluation report in outpatient rehabilitation for a patient who has had a stroke. Extract the information that is appropriate to include in the Intervention Plan section of the report. Rewrite this information under the appropriate headings in the space provided. The sentences should flow together smoothly.

1. Medical hx is significant for HTN.

2. Pt. will be instructed in self-stretching of right wrist and elbow.

3. Referral to orthotist to evaluate for specific AFO.

4. Pt. will be able to negotiate walking over 6-inch high obstacles.

5. Fx training to address balance and coordination during morning bathroom routine.

6. RLE strengthening exercises such as squats, stair stepping, and obstacle negotiation to improve standing and walking ability.

7. Discuss with patient options for long-distance mobility, including use of wheelchair.

8. Pt. will be seen 3×/wk for outpatient physical therapy, 45-min sessions.

9. Strength of right hip abductors will increase to 4/5.

10. Trng with appropriate assistive device (straight cane or quad cane) during ambulation indoors and outdoors, and transfers to improve safety, speed and distance.

11. Pt. will view video modeling strategies for improved UE function in patients who have had a stroke.

12. Pt. can ↑↓10 steps in 1 min 20 sec.

13. Pt. will be instructed in home walking program to improve speed and endurance; walking daily beginning with 10 min and progressing to 20 min over 4 wks.

Intervention plan: _____

_____

Coordination/communication: _____

_____

_____

Pt.-related instruction: _____

_____

_____

Procedural intervention: _____

_____

_____

Information that does not belong in this section (statement numbers): _____

Additional
Documentation Formats

CHAPTER 11

Documenting Daily Notes and Progress Notes: Elements of the SOAP Record

LEARNING OBJECTIVES

After reading this chapter and completing the exercises, the reader will be able to:

1. Identify and define the four components of a SOAP record.
2. Outline the components of writing daily notes and progress notes.
3. Appropriately document components of a daily note and progress note using a SOAP format.

Daily notes and progress notes are a key component of physical therapy documentation. In fact, many therapists spend a majority of their documentation time writing these types of notes. Although the focus of this book thus far has been on documenting the initial evaluation, all elements included in daily or progress notes are essentially components of the initial evaluation. The concepts discussed in the previous chapters all apply here.

The most commonly used format for writing daily notes is the SOAP note. The letters SOAP stand for subjective, objective, assessment, and plan. This format was discussed briefly in Chapter 2 and is presented here as a framework for daily note and progress note documentation. The SOAP note is a commonly used format and is one with which most medical personnel are familiar. With some modifications the SOAP note can provide the foundation for efficient, effective functional outcomes documentation in rehabilitation. This chapter presents a format for writing both daily notes and progress notes using the SOAP format.

DAILY NOTES

Daily or per session notes are written for each encounter a PT or PTA has with a patient. APTA Documen-

tation Guidelines (see Appendix A) outline the following components that should be included in each daily note:

- Patient self-report
- Identification of specific interventions provided, including frequency, intensity, and duration as appropriate
- Equipment provided
- Changes in patient status as they relate to the plan of care
- Adverse reaction to interventions, if any
- Factors that modify frequency or intensity of intervention
- Progression toward anticipated goals, including patient adherence to patient-related instructions
- Communication/consultation with providers, patient, family, and significant others

Although APTA Documentation Guidelines require documentation for each physical therapy encounter, the format of daily note documentation is at the discretion of each institution. Daily notes often are required for reimbursement purposes and must be provided as proof of service. Some facilities require a weekly progress note and relatively simple documentation on a per session basis.

CASE EXAMPLE 11-1	**DAILY NOTE DOCUMENTATION**

DAILY NOTE DOCUMENTATION
Setting: Outpatient

Name: Emily Rodriguez   *D.O.B.:* 2/3/70   *Date:* 1/5/02

Current Condition: 31 y.o. female 12-wks postpartum c̄ onset of stress incontinence p̄ vaginal delivery of first child.

GOAL

1. Decrease urine losses from 2 times daily to once per week.

S: Pt. reports urinary losses of 1 tablespoon have decreased to 1 × day over past 3 days. They occur primarily when coughing or during physical activities such as lifting baskets of laundry, running, and jumping. Pt. continues to wear 2 panty-liners daily as continued precaution to protect clothing.

O: Biofeedback re-assessment was completed in supine with noted improvement in EMG activity levels for pelvic muscle contractions. Fair strength of pelvic floor muscle contraction, held 5 sec × 7 reps. Pt. performed pelvic floor muscle contractions with the biofeedback program in the standing position. Additionally, pt. performed pelvic floor muscle contractions during a lunge to floor and back to standing, 3 reps each LE (practicing the movement for lifting a laundry basket). Pt. practiced performing pelvic muscle contractions prior to a cough, 5 reps. Pt. educated to perform a pelvic muscle contraction before cough or before lifting heavy objects to prevent incontinence. Revised home program to increase pelvic muscle contractions in sitting for 20 1-second contractions; followed by 20 minutes of 10-second contractions in sitting.

A: Pt. reports decrease in urinary losses over past 3 days, which correlates with observed improvements in EMG activity levels for pelvic floor muscle contractions. Pt. is responding well to intervention and home program.

P: Continue PT 1 ×/wk. Progress with pelvic muscle strength trng and muscle re-education during functional tasks, with instruction in progressive HEP to improve pt.'s level of ADLs.

Documentation of daily sessions can become unwieldy without some structure. The SOAP format is relatively easy to master and provides a quick format for writing a daily note. Specific components of SOAP note documentation for daily notes are listed in Figure 11-1. Examples of daily note documentation in different clinical settings are provided in Case Examples 11-1 and 11-2.

Goal(s)

In a functional outcomes report the SOAP format is modified so that the focus of the note is the functional outcome that the therapist was working toward in the particular treatment session. This is accomplished by adding a statement at the beginning of the SOAP note that identifies the functional goals that were the focus

of the treatment session. The goals written in this section typically are restatements of goals set at the time of the initial evaluation.

Common Pitfall Goals are not included. Restating the goal or goals forces the therapist to maintain a focus on the outcomes towards which therapeutic intervention is directed.

Subjective

In the subjective section of the note the therapist documents any statements or reports made by the patient, patient's family members or caregivers, or both. The purpose of this section is to detail the patient's own perception of his or her condition. This section of the note does not include direct observations made by the

Daily Note	
Goal(s)	List the functional and impairment goals that were addressed during this treatment session. If more than one, number them for easy identification.
Subjective (S)	Document any patient/client reports related to functional status (e.g., not just "pain", but how that pain interfered with functional activities) or disability (e.g., how improved functional activities are being integrated into patient's home or work life.)
Objective (O)	Outline treatments that were performed, including patient education and equipment provided. Include frequency, duration and intensity if appropriate. Indicate changes in patient's status, and any observed changes during or after treatment. Report any communication with providers or family members.
Assessment (A)	Indicate the progress that is being made towards the patient's goals. Discuss any factors that modify frequency or intensity of intervention and progression toward anticipated goals. Indicate any adverse responses by the patient to any intervention. Modify or set new goals if necessary.
Plan (P)	Indicate intervention plan for upcoming sessions. Report what patient will be doing between treatments (home program). Indicate what steps will be taken to reach functional goals.

FIGURE 11-1

Elements of daily note documentation using a SOAP format.

therapist. Therapists can report a patient's or caregiver's remarks in quotations if the exact phrasing is somehow pertinent. Documentation of subjective information should incorporate information that is relevant to the patient's progress in rehabilitation and specifically related to changes in functional performance or quality of life. It should not include extraneous information that is not directly related to the patient's current condition.

Common Pitfall   Therapist draws conclusions or passes judgment on a patient (e.g., *"Pt. over-reacting to symptoms"*). Therapist could also document nonpertinent information. For example, a therapist might write: *"Pt. reports she didn't like her last PT."* This statement is not pertinent.

Objective

The focus of the objective section is twofold: (1) to document the patient's progress toward the functional outcomes and (2) to provide details of the interventions performed. Therapists document the results of any tests and measures performed, specifically those that relate to achievement of the stated goal(s). Furthermore, the therapist specifies any procedural interventions that were performed, including location, frequency, intensity, duration, and/or repetitions, as appropriate.

Common Pitfall   Not enough detail is provided regarding specific interventions. Therapists may globally summarize the interventions performed in a daily note,

---

DOCUMENTING PAIN IN DAILY NOTES AND PROGRESS NOTES

Documentation of pain is often a critical component of daily note or progress note documentation. In the initial evaluation, a detailed description of pain is recommended, including location, quality, severity, timing, and factors that make it better or worse (see Box 7-1). The setting in which pain occurs, and any associated manifestations may also be included.

In the daily note or progress note documentation, a change in any component of pain is worthy of documentation. Decrease in pain severity (e.g., *"Pt. reports pain has decreased to 2/10 on VAS."*) or quality (e.g., *"Pt reports pain has gone from a burning, stabbing pain to an aching pain."*) can be significant indicators

of patient improvement. Thus it is not essential in the daily note or progress note to completely re-document the detailed pain assessment provided in an initial note. Rather, changes in the patient's report of pain should be specifically documented.

Reports of pain (because they are inherently subjective) should typically be documented in the subjective section of a daily note or a progress note. However, if report of pain is incidental to an objective statement, then it can be included in the objective section, e.g., *"Pt. performed 10 reps × 3 sets SLR with no increase in pain."* This statement's focus is on the intervention being performed.

---

such as: *"E-stim"* or *"MH"* or *"Ther ex."* Instead, specific details should be provided for each intervention performed: *"Ther ex included seated knee extension through full range, 30 lbs, 8 reps × 3; prone knee flexion through full range, 20 lbs, 10 reps × 3."* It is often useful to use flowcharts to document such information.

Assessment

In the Assessment section, the therapist provides an analysis of the patient's progress, including reasons why the patient is or is not improving as expected. The therapist summarizes the patient's progress and discusses those factors contributing to or hindering progress. The patient's overall response to the intervention should also be discussed in this section.

Common Pitfall The Assessment is too vague and not meaningful. Avoid vague terms like *"Pt. tol Rx well"* or *"Pt. is improving."* Such statements provide little insight into the effectiveness of the intervention. A better example would be: *"Pt. has demonstrated improved tolerance to performing ther. ex regime and has reported an increase in sitting tolerance time at work".*

Plan

The final section of the daily note outlines the plan. Any specific interventions for upcoming sessions should be documented, including any changes in the intervention strategy.

Common Pitfall The upcoming plan is not documented. Documentation such as "Cont Rx," while sometimes appropriate, provides no information about how the

therapist plans to continue to progress the patient. A better example would be: *"Increase number of repetitions in squatting and wall slide exercises to 20."* As the therapist reviews the patient's record at the next visit, this statement will serve as a reminder as to the intended plan.

Legal Issues

Daily note documentation is critical for legal purposes. If issues or conflicts arise, the daily notes will be highly scrutinized. Thus therapists should dedicate appropriate time to clear and effective documentation on a per session basis. "A poorly documented patient/client record can serve as powerful evidence in support of a suit, even when the accusations are frivolous" (Lewis, 2002).

Below are some important documentation guidelines for daily or per session notes, adapted from Lewis (2002):

1. Timeliness. Therapists should write daily notes as soon as possible after a session. This helps keep information fresh in their minds and minimizes the chance of errors.
2. Decision-making rationale. Each section should flow logically from the next, and the therapist's decisions about assessment, goals, and intervention should be supported by concrete data.
3. Patient/client behavior. Missed or canceled appointments must be documented in the patient's medical record. For example, *"Pt. called at 9:00 AM to cancel 1:30 pm appt. Pt. reports his L shoulder was sore from doing too much lifting yesterday. Next appt scheduled in 2 days."* This provides the time the appointment was canceled, detailed information as to the reason the

CASE EXAMPLE 11-2

DAILY NOTE DOCUMENTATION
Setting: Inpatient Rehabilitation

Name: Wally Narcessian   *D.O.B.:* 3/7/30   *Date:* 6/20/02 (10:26:00 AM)

Current Condition: COPD/pneumonia

GOALS

1. Pt. will demonstrate productive cough in a seated position, 3/4 trials.
2. Pt. will ambulate 150 ft with supervision, no A device, on level indoor surfaces.

S: Pt. reports not feeling well today, "I'm very tired."

O: Auscultation findings: scattered rhonchi all lung fields. Chest PT was performed in sitting (ant and post). Techniques included percussion, vibration, and shaking. Pt. performed a weak combined abdominal and upper costal cough that was nonbronchospastic, congested, and nonproductive. The cough/huff was performed with VC. Pectoral stretch/thoracic cage mobilizations performed in seated position. Pt. given towel roll placed in back of seat to open up ant chest wall. Strengthening exercises in standing—pt. performed hip flexion, extension, and abduction; knee flexion 10 reps × 1 set B. Pt. performs HEP with supervision (in evenings with wife). Pt. instructed to hold tissue over trach when speaking to prevent infection and explained importance of drinking enough water.

A: Pt. continues to present with congestion and limitations in coughing productivity. Pt. has been compliant with evening exercise program, which has resulted in increased tol to therapeutic exercise regime and an increase in LE strength. Amb. not attempted today 2° to pt. report of fatigue. Pt. should be able to tolerate short distance ambulation within the next few days.

P: Cont. current treatment plan including CPT; emphasize productive coughing techniques; increase strengthening exer reps to 15; attempt amb again tomorrow.

appointment was canceled, and information about future appointments.

4. Prior and concurrent treatment. Therapists should document any other interventions a patient is currently undergoing, or has undergone in the past. For example, "*Pt. reports he has begun acupuncture 2 ×/week to facilitate back pain relief.*"

5. Telephone conversations. Any conversations pertinent to the patient and the rehabilitation program should be documented. Such documentation should include the name, time, issues discussed, and the resolution or action. For example: "*PT called pt.'s orthopedic surgeon, Dr. Smith, to discuss pt.'s report of increased pain in L ankle at fracture site. MD stated to D/C PT immediately and refer pt. back to him for evaluation.*"

6. Informed consent and referral. Documentation of informed consent in an initial evaluation is discussed in Chapter 10. In a daily note, informed consent should be documented if changes to the plan of care are being implemented. For example, the following could be documented relative to the above example: "*Pt. was informed of phone conversation and MD's orders and was instructed to call MD immediately for an appt. Pt. agreed to this and stated he would call MD upon returning home.*"

7. Adverse incidents. Therapists should follow their institution's guidelines for documenting of an adverse incident. Typically, this is done on an incident report. Therapists should document in the medical record only pertinent clinical findings and indicate that a report has been filed.

CASE EXAMPLE 11-3

PROGRESS NOTE DOCUMENTATION
Setting: Outpatient

Name: Melissa Chau   *D.O.B.:* 12/26/75   *Date:* 10/01/01

Current Condition: Patellofemoral dysfunction, 1 wk reevaluation

GOALS

1. Ascend and descend 2 flights of stairs, pain free.
2. Run on level surfaces 2 miles in 20 minutes, 2 × week, pain free.

S: "My knee is hurting less when I'm not walking." (0/10 on VAS)

O: Rx as per flow sheet. *Ambulation/stair climbing:* Pt. able to walk 1/2 mile at comfortable speed (65 m/min). Able to ascend 2 flights of stairs pain free. Pain rated as 4/10 (sharp pain) descending 1 flight of stairs. *Running:* Pt. has not yet engaged in running activity. *Strength:* L quadriceps: 4/5 L hamstrings: 5/5; R quads and hamstrings: 5/5. *Left unilateral stance time, static:* 20 sec. *Right unilateral stance time, static:* 60 sec.

A: Pt. is exhibiting a steady improvement in eccentric control of left quadriceps when descending stairs, indicated by an increase in control of descent and a decrease in reported pain. Patellar taping techniques are being used to recruit left vastus medialis. Balance deficits are still apparent indicated by limited unilateral stance time on the left. Steady progress is being made toward the goal of pain-free stairs negotiation. Continued strength and balance gains are necessary for the patient to achieve the second goal related to running. Cross-training has been emphasized as well, with cycling being introduced to the pt.'s routine.

P: Continue current exercise regime, with progression in reps and weight as tolerated. Home program, which consists of SLRs, squats, and step-ups, is to be completed daily. Physical therapy sessions will continue 2 × week to include low impact activities (e.g., jogging on trampoline). Eval for orthotics next session.

EXERCISE FLOW SHEET

Name: Chau, Melissa, 2001

Modality/ Procedure	Date		
	9-27-01	9-28-01	10-1-01
Eval/Treatment Number	1	2	3
Evaluation	√		
Patellar taping (L)		Medial glide	Medial glide
Patellar mobilizations (L)		Medial glide	Medial glide
Ice (at end of Rx)		10 minutes	10 minutes
EXERCISES			
Lateral step-ups		4 inch, 2 × 10	4 inch, 3 × 10
Chair squats		0# 3 × 10	0# 3 × 15
SLRs	0# 3 × 10	0# 3 × 15	1# 3 × 10
Left unilateral stance		L: 25 sec	L: 30 sec
Leg press		B:80# L:40# 3 × 10	B:80# L:40# 3 × 15
Stretching (ITB, quad/hamstrings/calf)	3 × 30 sec	3 × 30 sec	3 × 30 sec

PROGRESS NOTES

Progress notes are written to provide an update of a patient's status; these notes often are based on a reexamination. A progress note can have a similar format to an initial evaluation, and the functional outcomes framework presented in earlier chapters can be used. However, the SOAP format can also be utilized. Case Examples 11-3 and 11-4 provide sample documentation of progress notes using a SOAP format.

Figure 11-2 outlines the key elements of each section of the progress note based on a SOAP format. Progress notes should be succinct and easy to read, because they often are used by third-party payers to justify the need for skilled therapeutic intervention. Comparisons of pre-intervention and post-intervention functional performance are especially useful. Also, therapists should document any interventions that were performed during the reevaluation period and provide justification for the need for continued therapy.

The progress note typically covers multiple visits and therefore provides a summary of the patient's progress to date. The following are key elements of a progress note or reevaluation report:

- The patient's progress toward the stated goals must be clearly stated with revision of goals as needed.

	Progress Note
Goal(s)	List the functional goals that were addressed during the reevaluation time period.
Subjective (S)	Summarize patient reports related to changes in function or disability, progress toward goals or intervention plan.
Objective (O)	List re-tests of the patient's functional abilities. If functional abilities are improving, quantify the improvement (e.g., "*increase in tolerance for standing at workbench from 30 seconds to 2 min*"). Include results of the physical examination or observations of impairments as they relate to the functional progress. Summarize skilled interventions that were performed, including education. Describe the patient's response to intervention and improvement from the previous period.
Assessment (A)	Discuss to what extent the functional goals have been achieved, and if not, why not. Summarize observations of how impairments relate to the functional progress (revision of PT diagnosis). Discuss why continued PT intervention will address these problems. Modify goals or set new goals.
Plan (P)	Indicate modifications or changes to the treatment plan specified at the onset of care.

FIGURE 11-2

Elements of progress note documentation using a SOAP format.

CASE EXAMPLE 11-4

PROGRESS NOTE DOCUMENTATION
Setting: Outpatient clinic setting

Name: Ralph Fisher   *D.O.B.:* 12/19/55   *Date:* 7/8/01

Current Condition: Huntington's disease (HD) × 11 yrs; 1 mo reevaluation

GOALS (12 WKS)

1. Pt. will experience no falls during indoor or outdoor ambulation, over a 12-wk period.
2. Pt. will increase average outdoor walking speed on sidewalk with use of cane to 50 m/min, for distances greater than 400 m.
3. Pt. will be independent in performing home exercise program.

S: Pt. reports that his balance "is getting better" and that he has had no falls in past 4 wks (since initial evaluation). He reports that he is not yet comfortable using the cane for outdoor ambulation. He reports having some difficulty keeping up with walking and turning exercises on exercise videotape.

O: Pt. has been seen 1 ×/wk for 4 wks to address balance impairments and ambulation difficulties related to HD. Intervention has consisted of (1) gait training on indoor and outdoor surfaces, including safety instruction and strategies to improve gait speed; (2) balance exercises and balance training in standing, emphasizing improving proactive balance; instruction in home program with exercise videotape (35 min in length)—exercises include ROM/flexibility, strengthening, and cardiovascular; discussion of home safety and recommendations made for grab bars in bathroom, removal of rugs, and supportive chair for mealtimes. A summary of pt.'s current functional abilities and impairments is provided below.

Functional Abilities: Pt. is able to walk indoors s̄ A device; avg. walking speed 42 m/min. Pt. ambulates outdoors on sidewalk with slower gait speed (35 m/min) and is very cautious. Pt. avoids stairs and uneven surfaces whenever possible due to fear of falling; these activities have not yet been assessed in therapy. Activities of Balance Confidence (indicative of balance confidence during various functional tasks) remains at 80% (100% = complete confidence). Continues to demonstrate LOB (to the R and posteriorly) during indoor and outdoor ambulation but has I recovery.

Impairments: *Dystonia:* unchanged; mod. trunk dystonia resulting in posturing into extension and R lateral flexion; *Chorea:* unchanged; mod. chorea × 4 extremities; *Balance:* Berg Balance Scale score increased from 39 to 44; pt. improved in tandem stance, turning in place, and picking up object from floor. Single limb stance unchanged; limited to <2 sec B.

A: Pt. has demonstrated improvements in balance as measured by the Berg Balance Scale and has not had any falls in a 4-wk period. Pt. is able to perform HEP program independently with modifications. Pt. requires continued PT to address slow walking speed (Goal 2) and standing balance impairments, focusing on single limb stance to continue to minimize falls risk (Goal 1).

P: (1) Gait training indoors and outdoors to address safety, speed, and balance (proactive and reactive). (2) Balance training exercises, emphasizing single limb stance activities. (3) Revision of home program to modify walking and turning activities so pt. can keep up with tape. (4) Cont. education re: use of straight cane during outdoor ambulation. (5) Evaluate stair climbing, curb negotiation, and uneven surface ambulation, and initiate training for functional benefit, balance improvement, and strengthening.

- Evidence should be provided that skilled intervention was required to achieve the stated goals (particularly important for Medicare documentation, see Chapter 12).
- The plan of care should be revised as needed, with justification for continued therapy.

SUMMARY

- Daily notes and progress notes can be organized as a functional outcomes report using a SOAP format.

- Documentation is required for every physical therapy encounter and should include information about the interventions provided and progress toward stated goals.

- Daily notes are important legal records. Therapists should carefully document all aspects directly pertinent to patient's current physical therapy intervention and his or her current condition.

- Progress notes provide an update of a patient's status. Progress toward the stated goals is discussed and justification for continued therapy is provided.

EXERCISE 11-1

The following statements could be written as part of daily SOAP notes. Using Figure 11-2, classify each of the following statements into their appropriate category based in the SOAP format: G = Goal; S = Subjective; O = Objective; A = Assessment; P = Plan.

SOAP Statement	SOAP Section G, S, O, A, or P
1. Performed 10 reps SLR B.	_____
2. Pt. reports she was able to walk with her daughter out to get the mail yesterday and did not experience any dizziness.	_____
3. Treatment next session will include progression to stationary bike × 10 min.	_____
4. Pt. walked 15 ft from bed to bathroom without SOB in 30 sec.	_____
5. Pt. states that she "felt sore" after last treatment session.	_____
6. Pt. is progressing well with increasing repetitions of LE strengthening exercises and has achieved goal #1.	_____
7. Pitting edema noted in R ankle.	_____
8. Pt. was instructed to continue to maintain R leg in elevated position while sitting at desk during the day.	_____
9. Pt. will transfer from bed to wheelchair independently, 4/5 trials within 2 wks.	_____
10. Pt. states she is anxious to return to work.	_____
11. Pt. will continue with daily walking program at home during off-therapy days, progressing to 20 min each day by next wk.	_____
12. Pt. will stand s̄ A for up to 1 min within 1 wk.	_____
13. Pt. reports pain in low back while walking as 5/10 on VAS and 8/10 while sitting at desk at work.	_____
14. Pt's. fear of falling is limiting his progress in improving his ability to ambulate in crowded environments and outdoors.	_____
15. Pt. reports that she is going back to work on a trial basis next week.	_____

EXERCISE 11-2

Identify whether the following statements belong in the SUBJECTIVE or OBJECTIVE section of either a daily or progress SOAP note. Identify the errors in each statement. Errors could include: not enough detail, too much detail, not appropriate, or negative connotation. Indicate the specific word or words that are problematic, if applicable. Rewrite a more appropriate statement in the space provided.

Statement	Subjective or Objective	What Is Wrong?	Rewrite
EXAMPLE: Mr. Jones reports that he has been unable to do anything.	Subjective	Not enough detail; unclear as to what "anything" is referring to.	Mr. Jones reports that he is unable to play the organ at church and give music lessons due to the pain in his L elbow.
1. Pt. states he hates using his walker.			
2. Pt. says she is so much happier with the care she is receiving at this facility. She was disgusted with her previous medical care; she feels the doctors and therapists were completely noncaring and didn't know what they were doing.			
3. Pt. has an awkward gait.			
4. PROM at the knee is getting better.			
5. Pt. is very confused.			
6. Pt. reports that his son is concerned.			
7. Pt. c/o fatigue after walking for 5 min.			

Statement	Subjective or Objective	What Is Wrong?	Rewrite
8. Timmy has difficulty keeping his head up for prolonged periods.	_____	_____	_____
9. Pt. complains of pain in left shoulder.	_____	_____	_____
10. Pt. performed 10 reps of knee exercises.	_____	_____	_____

EXERCISE 11-3

The following statements are taken from various sections of a daily SOAP note written in an acute rehabilitation facility for a patient who had third-degree burns of his LEs. Rewrite the information in the space below under the appropriate SOAP heading (Goals, Subjective, Objective, Assessment, Plan). All statements can be categorized under one of these headings. The sentences should flow together smoothly.

1. ROM B hip flexion will increase to 0-120°.

2. 6 minute walk test—1200′ without assistive device; HR changed from 80 bpm to 120 bpm.

3. Consult with MD this afternoon re: expected x-ray results of L ankle.

4. Pt. has made notable improvement in B hip flexion AROM, which is resulting in improvements in reaching and lifting abilities, and transitions to floor.

5. Pt ↑↓ 3 flights (12 stairs) of 8″ steps independently, using SOS pattern to ascend, and R rail to descend, SOS; HR ↑ to 120 bpm.

6. Pt. reports L heel/ankle pain continues; pain at rest in morning 2/10, increases to 5/10 in the afternoon and evening.

7. Practiced reaching activities in standing, including picking up objects of various weight and height from floor with emphasis on controlled movements and maintaining proper body mechanics.

8. Continue with current Tx plan, with emphasis on soft tissue mobilization, LE flexibility, transitional skills, and improving ambulation and stair climbing ability.

9. Pt. will amb. 2000′ in 6 minutes independently, negotiating uneven outdoor terrain, HR <110 bpm.

10. Hip flexion AROM R: 0-110°; L: 0-95°.

11. Inspection of wound lateral and posterior aspect of L thigh, reapplied bacitracin, adaptic, and padding to blisters.

12. Pt. independently performed self-stretching of bilateral gastroc/soleus and hamstrings while sitting on floor; hip flexor stretch in side-lying position (30 sec hold, 3 times each).

13. Pt. continues to improve 6-minute walk test and stand←→floor mobility; awaiting x-ray results of L ankle due to pt.'s report of persistent L ankle/heel pain.

14. Pt. will independently perform transitions stand←→floor.

15. Pt. required min A to transfer from stand to kneeling and kneeling to long sitting.

SOAP DOCUMENTATION

G _____

_____

_____

_____

S _____

_____

_____

_____

O _____

_____

_____

_____

A _____

_____

_____

_____

P _____

_____

_____

_____

CHAPTER 12

Specialized Documentation

LEARNING OBJECTIVES

After reading this chapter and completing the exercises, the reader will be able to:

1. List the essential features of a discharge summary.
2. Describe the essential components of documentation for Medicare reimbursement.
3. Discuss the Medicare guidelines for documenting skilled therapy services.
4. Identify the key elements of letters to insurance companies that will help to maximize reimbursement.
5. Identify the key components of documentation in early intervention and school-based settings.

Physical therapy documentation can take many different forms. This book has focused on documentation of the initial evaluation, as well as progress notes and daily notes (see Chapter 11). However, PTs write many other types of documentation ranging from Medicare forms, letters to insurance companies, and individualized service plans (IEPs). This chapter discusses specific issues related to some of the most common forms of specialized documentation and presents a framework for easy integration of a functional outcomes approach into each form.

Another important component of a discharge summary is an overview of the patient's progress relative to the stated goals from the initial evaluation. The interventions used should also be outlined. Importantly, the therapist should discuss the plan for the patient at this point. This plan may include a home program, or if the patient has moved to another facility (e.g., discharge from acute care to a skilled nursing facility), then any recommendations for continued therapy or other services should be provided.

DISCHARGE SUMMARIES

At the completion of an episode of care, therapists typically write a discharge summary. The main purpose of a discharge summary is to document the status of the patient at the time he or she is discharged. A discharge summary does not require a complete reevaluation. However, therapists should report changes in the functional limitations and impairments that are pertinent to the stated goals. These can be provided in a summary statement or in a table.

PATIENT EDUCATION MATERIALS

An important set of tools used by PTs are patient education materials and home programs. This practice occurs in all types of settings and patient populations and is one of the cornerstones of physical therapy intervention. Written instructions must be completed carefully, with specific attention directed to the patient's educational level, language capabilities, and learning style. Whenever possible, pictures or graphical information can be very helpful to provide a visual representation of the information being conveyed.

Many different types of patient education materials are available for purchase through various organizations. Many can be tailored to individual patient needs. For example, many materials are available with exercise prescription "boxes" containing hundreds of exercises that can be photocopied. The number of computer software packages designed with this same purpose has increased. Therapists should also be sure to place a copy of any patient education materials in the patient's medical record, including the date and additional verbal instructions provided.

MEDICARE

Key Elements of Documentation

Medicare is the federal health insurance plan for individuals age 65 and older. Individuals with a permanent disability also receive Medicare benefits. Thus Medicare is one of the most common reimbursement mechanisms for PTs.

The Center for Medicare and Medicaid Services (CMS), a government agency, contracts with different insurance companies (called Medicare *carriers* or *intermediaries*) to manage and implement Medicare benefits (Vance, 2002). These intermediaries require specific documentation to ensure reimbursement. The following are essential components that should be documented by the PT for the initial evaluation. Each component has been explained in detail in other chapters in this book.

- Technical information, such as patient's age, date of birth (DOB), primary diagnosis (International Classification of Disease [ICD]-9 code), facility and patient identification numbers
- Date of onset
- Medical history
- Reason for therapy intervention
- Current status
- Plan of treatment
- Goals

In some cases, specific forms are recommended by Medicare intermediaries to provide a standardized format for documentation. For example, the Health Care Financing Administration (HCFA) 700—Plan of Treatment for Outpatient Rehabilitation is a standardized format for the initial evaluation and progress note at the end of a billing period for patients receiving services in skilled nursing facilities and outpatient settings. Figure 12-1 provides an example of documentation using HCFA 700. As shown in this example, a functional outcomes approach can readily be incorporated into Medicare documentation. (If all pertinent information is included on the HCFA 700 form, no other documentation is necessary.)

Because guidelines for Medicare documentation change frequently, therapists working with patients with Medicare coverage should consult the Centers for Medicare and Medicaid services (CMS) website (www.cms.gov) for updated information on Medicare and Medicaid documentation.

Prospective Payment

Prospective payment systems are used in home health agencies, skilled nursing facilities, and rehabilitation hospitals as a means to manage escalating Medicare costs in these settings. The CMS has developed different patient classifications systems for each of these settings. These classifications are determined by specialized documentation completed by medical personnel to categorize the patient according to various functional and medical factors, depending on the setting. The Minimum Data Set (MDS), Outcome and Assessment and Information Set (OASIS), and the Inpatient Rehabilitation Facility Patient Assessment Instrument (IRF-PAI) are the assessment instruments used in skilled nursing facilities, home health agencies, and inpatient rehabilitation, respectively. Figure 12-2 provides a description of each of these tools.

The involvement of therapists in completing these tools varies depending on the institution or agency. Some institutions require PTs to complete portions of these tools, such as the mobility section, and others require nursing staff to complete the entire assessment. These tools use numerical ratings rather than narrative reporting, and extensive training is typically provided. If computerized documentation is used in a practice setting, these forms can be completed more easily and integrated into institution-specific documentation formats (see Chapter 13 for examples of computerized documentation using standardized assessment tools).

Daily Notes

Medicare reimbursement relies on documentation as its primary (if not only) source of determining whether a claim is paid or denied. Thus therapists must be very diligent about their documentation to appropriately reflect the patient's status. All of the issues discussed in Chapter 11 related to daily notes are applicable for Medicare documentation. Although current Medicare guidelines state that progress needs to be documented at least monthly (except for home health care, which is 60 days), no specific guideline is required for documentation of daily notes. Vance (2002) suggests that daily notes are a critical part of Medicare documentation.

DEPARTMENT OF HEALTH AND HUMAN SERVICES
HEALTH CARE FINANCING ADMINISTRATION

FORM APPROVED
OMB NO. 0938-0227

PLAN OF TREATMENT FOR OUTPATIENT REHABILITATION (COMPLETE FOR INITIAL CLAIMS ONLY)

1. PATIENT'S LAST NAME TEST	FIRST NAME M.I. TEST	2. PROVIDER NO.	3. HICN
4. PROVIDER NAME	5. MEDICAL RECORD NO. (*Optional*)	6. ONSET DATE 8/1/2002 12:00:00AM	7. SOC. DATE 8/15/2002 12:00:00AM

8. TYPE [X] PT [ ] OT [ ] SLP [ ] CR [ ] RT [ ] PS [ ] SN [ ] SW

9. PRIMARY DIAGNOSIS Hip Fracture; s/p ORIF	10. TREATMENT DIAGNOSIS Decr. functional ability and pain	11. VISITS FROM SOC. 6

12. PLAN OF TREATMENT FUNCTIONAL GOALS

GOALS (Short Term): 2 wks

AROM GOAL: Patient will obtain 90 degrees of hip flexion and 0 degrees of hip extension on the right.
AMBULATION GOAL: Patient will ambulate 500 feet with a straight cane with supervision on level / indoor surfaces .
CURB GOAL: Patient will negotiate a 4" curb with SC and contact guard of 1.
STAIR GOAL: Patient will be able to negotiate 10 steps (7") using a step to step ascending pattern and step to step descending pattern with supervision and one rail.
PAIN GOAL: Decrease resting pain level to 2/10
BALANCE GOAL: Patient will be able to pick up small object off the floor (less than 3 lbs.) maintaining good balance and hip precautions.

OUTCOME (Long Term): At time of discharge

AMBULATION GOAL: Patient will ambulate 750 feet with a straight cane independently on all surfaces (indoor and outdoor).
STAIR GOAL: Patient will be able to negotiate 15 steps (7") using a step over step ascending pattern and step over step descending pattern independently and a straight cane and one rail.
CURB GOAL: Patient will negotiate a (4") standard curb with a straight cane independently.
ENDURANCE GOAL: 6 Minute Walk - Patient will be able to ambulate 450 feet in 6 minutes.
HEP GOAL: Pt. will be Indep. with home exercise program.

PLAN

Therapeutic Activity - AROM, PROM and strengthening to (R) hip musculature
Gait Training - To increase safety, distance and endurance
Therapeutic Procedure - stationary bicycle, treadmill
Patient Education/HEP Instruction - Continued hip precautions, standing and supine LE strengthening, and standing balance exercises

13. SIGNATURE (*professional establishing POC including prof. designation*)

14. FREQ/DURATION (e.g. 3/Wk x 4 Wk.)

3x/week for 4 weeks

I CERTIFY THE NEED FOR THESE SERVICES FURNISHED UNDER THIS PLAN OF TREATMENT AND WHILE UNDER MY CARE   [ ] N/A

15. PHYSICIAN'S SIGNATURE | **16. DATE**

17. CERTIFICATION
FROM 8/15/2002 12:00:0THROUGH   8/31/2002 12:00:00 [ ] N/A

18. ON FILE (*Print/type physician's name*)
[ ]

20. INITIAL ASSESSMENT (*History, medical complications, level of function at start of care. Reason for referral*)

19. PRIOR HOSPITALIZATION
FROM 8/1/2002 12:00:00A THROUGH   8/10/2002 12:00:00 [ ] N/A

Patient is a 71 y/o female who tripped over her cat and fell. The fall resulted in a (R) hip fx. requiring an ORIF. Following acute care hospitalization, the patient returned home with continuing OP services.
Pt reports pain in the right anterior hip/groin with a post surgical onset. Pain is described as dull and stiff with an intermittent pattern. The primary factor that aggravates the condition is prolonged ambulation, stair negotiation, and prolonged standing . The primary factor that relieves the patient's symtoms is rest and medication.
PAIN: Current pain level is 4/10
AROM: (R) Hip extension −10 degrees; (R) hip flexion 10-75 degrees
PROM: (R) Hip extension −5 degrees; (R) hip flexion 5-80 degrees
AMBULATION STATUS: Patient amb. 150 ft with a straight cane and supervision of 1 person on indoor/level surfaces. Patient requires contact guard on outdoor surfaces for 100 feet, with min A on curbs and ramps.
STAIR NEGOTIATION: Patient requires contact guard of 1 to negotiate 8 (7") stairs and reports increase in pain (6/10) during descending stairs.

21. FUNCTIONAL LEVEL (*at end of billing period*) **PROGRESS REPORT**   [X] CONTINUE SERVICES OR   [ ] DC SERVICES

Patient has made significant improvements in the following areas: Ambulation - patient can ambulate 500 feet with SC and supervision with occasional loss of balance with ind. recovery; pt. can amb on outdoor surfaces including grass and sidewalks with a SC and supervision. Stairs - patient negotiates 10 (7") stairs with supervison using S-T-S pattern. Patient now reports pain level during activity to be 2/10. AROM: (R) hip extension 0 degrees, (R) hip flexion -5 to 90 degrees. PROM: (R) hip extension 5 degrees, (R) hip flexion 0 to 100 degrees.
Proactive and reactive standing balance is limited (BERG BALANCE score 43/56—placing patient at risk for falls).

22. SERVICE DATES
FROM 8/1/2002   THROUGH 8/31/2002

FORM HCFA-700 (11-91)

FIGURE 12-1

Sample Medicare HCFA Form 700 completed in an outpatient rehabilitation setting.

FORM	SETTING/POPULATION	DESCRIPTION
Inpatient Rehabilitation Facility–Patient Assessment Instrument (IRF-PAI)	Inpatient rehabilitation; prospective payment system	Uses FIM scores and comorbidities to classify patients into specific case-mix groups and payment categories.
Minimum Data Set–Resource utilization groups (MDS–RUGS)	Nursing home; skilled nursing facilities	Comprehensive assessment of patient's functional status and medical condition; used to categorize patients into resource utilization groupings to determine the amount of payment.
Outcome and Assessment and Information Set (OASIS)	Home health agencies	Measures outcomes in home health care and determines reimbursement for services.

FIGURE 12-2

Each of these regulatory forms are used to categorize patients for reimbursement purposes. Computerized documentation of the physical therapy notes and other medical record can improve the coordination with such forms and minimize redundancy of recording the information.

A reviewer is unable to determine whether specific interventions are reimbursable without daily documentation. A grid format or flow sheet covering several days of interventions can be used, but it should include information indicating (1) the skilled intervention that was performed and (2) progress toward the stated goals and any major changes in the patient's condition. Documentation of provision of skilled intervention by a PT is a key component that is evaluated by Medicare reviewers. Reviewers look for evidence that the intervention could have been provided by other nonskilled personnel. Figure 12-3 provides an outline of the guidelines that can be used to determine whether a service is "skilled."

Progress Notes

Progress notes written for Medicare are called *recertifications*. These progress notes are required to help Medicare reviewers determine whether the services provided are reimbursable. The progress note contains many of the same components of the initial evaluation, including the following (Vance, 2002):

- Patient and facility identification number
- Date of birth
- Primary diagnosis and therapy diagnosis, and ICD 9 codes
- Number of visits from start of care
- Certification dates
- Start of care date
- Date of onset
- Rehabilitation potential
- Discussion of progress or lack of progress and justification of need for continued skilled therapy or discharge, if appropriate
- Intervention plan
- Short-term and long-term goals
- Frequency and duration

HCFA Form 701 (updated plan of progress for outpatient rehabilitation) is a standard form typically used in outpatient settings and skilled nursing facilities. Figure 12-4 provides an example of a completed 701 form using a functional outcomes format. This form can be used as both a progress note and a discharge summary form. Blank 700 and 701 forms can be found in Appendix D.

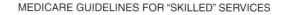

MEDICARE GUIDELINES FOR "SKILLED" SERVICES

- The complexity of the services rendered is such that it can only be safely and effectively carried out by, or under the supervision of, a skilled PT.

- The nature of the service, or skills required for safe and effective delivery of that service, requires the skills of licensed rehabilitation personnel, such as a PT.

- The patient's medical condition is a valid factor in considering skilled need, but his/her diagnosis or prognosis should never be the sole factor in deciding whether a service is skilled or not.

- A deciding factor as to whether or not a patient requires the skills of a PT is not the patient's potential for recovery, but whether the patient requires the skills of a PT versus nonskilled personnel.

- A service that is not ordinarily considered skilled could be considered skilled in the presence of a special medical complication that requires a PT to perform a procedure or supervise or observe the service in question.

- The total condition and complexity of the patient requires skilled management of the services provided even though many or all of the specific services are unskilled.

FIGURE 12-3

Guidelines used by Medicare to determine whether or not a service is "skilled." These components must be reflected in physical therapy documentation, specifically the initial evaluation.

Adapted from Vance TN: *Medicare guidelines explained for the physical therapist: a practical resource guide for physical therapy service delivery,* Gaylord, Mich, 2002, National Rehabilitation Services.

LETTERS TO JUSTIFY SERVICES OR EQUIPMENT

Therapists are commonly required to provide justification for the services or equipment they provide or plan to provide. Letters of medical necessity are often required for purchases of expensive medical equipment, such as customized wheelchairs, particularly those being purchased through the Medicaid system. Such letters must provide detailed information about the nature of the patient's problems and current medical status, and the specific benefits the patient will receive from the particular equipment (a sample letter is shown in Figure 12-5). If special components or additions above and beyond standard equipment are required, each item should be separately and explicitly justified.

Therapists also frequently write letters to request approval for additional PT visits, or reimbursement for services after a claim has been denied. In these situations, therapists should include specific objective data outlining (1) the functional progress the patient has made in therapy to date, using objective and standardized tests whenever possible; and (2) an overview of the specific skilled therapy intervention that the patient received (or will receive) and rationale for each intervention (Figure 12-6). Tables, charts, grids, or bulleted lists are very useful in demonstrating progress in therapy and are more readable for reviewers who see many files each day.

When available, therapists should provide reviewers and insurance companies with current literature or research reports to support the use of a particular intervention for a patient or patient population. This can be in the form of an entire article, which is sent with a detailed letter, or a summary of a research article cited in the body of the letter.

Therapists must take care to ensure the letters are easy to read, use correct spelling and grammar, are readable, and avoid the use of jargon terms. Although these factors apply to all forms of documentation, they are particularly important for letters to insurance companies. Although therapists should not oversimplify their documentation, they should use terminology that can be relatively easily understood and should define any terminology that is unlikely to be known.

DEPARTMENT OF HEALTH AND HUMAN SERVICES
HEALTH CARE FINANCING ADMINISTRATION

FORM APPROVED
OMB NO. 0938-0227

UPDATED PLAN OF PROGRESS FOR OUTPATIENT REHABILITATION
(Complete for Interim to Discharge Claims, Photocopy of HCFA-700 or 701 is required)

1. PATIENT'S LAST NAME	FIRST NAME	M.I.	2. PROVIDER NO.	3. HICN
TEST	TEST			

4. PROVIDER NAME	5. MEDICAL RECORD NO. (*Optional*)	6. ONSET DATE	7. SOC. DATE
		8/1/2002 12:00:00AM	8/15/2002 12:00:00AM

8. TYPE	9. PRIMARY DIAGNOSIS	10. TREATMENT DIAGNOSIS	11. VISITS FROM SOC.
[X] PT [ ] OT [ ] SLP [ ] CR	Hip Fracture; s/p ORIF	Decr. functional ability and pain	12
[ ] RT [ ] PS [ ] SN [ ] SW	12. FREQ/DURATION (e.g. 3/Wk x 4 Wk.) 3x/week for 4 weeks		

13. CURRENT PLAN UPDATE TREATMENT FUNCTIONAL GOALS (*Specifiy changes to goals and plan*)

GOALS (Short Term): 2 wks

AROM GOAL: Patient will obtain 90 degrees of hip flexion and 0 degrees of hip extension on the right.
CURB GOAL: Patient will negotiate a 4" curb with SC and contact guard of 1.
BALANCE GOAL: Patient will be able to pick up small object off the floor (less than 3 lbs.) maintaining good balance and hip precautions.

OUTCOME (Long Term): At time of discharge

AMBULATION GOAL: Patient will ambulate 750 feet with a straight cane independently on all surfaces (indoor and outdoor).
STAIR GOAL: Patient will be able to negotiate 15 steps (7") using a step over step ascending pattern and step over step descending pattern independently and a straight cane and one rail.
CURB GOAL: Patient will negotiate a (4") standard curb with a straight cane independently.
ENDURANCE GOAL: 6 Minute Walk - Patient will be able to ambulate 450 feet in 6 minutes.
HEP GOAL: Pt. will be Indep. with home exercise program.

PLAN

Therapeutic Activity - AROM, PROM and strengthening to (R) hip musculature
Gait Training - To increase safety, distance and endurance
Therapeutic Procedure - stationary bicycle, treadmill
Patient Education/HEP Instruction - Continued hip precautions, standing and supine LE strengthening, and standing balance exercises

I HAVE REVIEWED THIS PLAN OF TREATMENT AND RECERTIFY A CONTINUING NEED FOR SERVICES

15. PHYSICIAN'S SIGNATURE

16. DATE

14. RECERTIFICATION
FROM 09/01/2002 THROUGH 09/13/2002

17. ON FILE (*Print/type physician's name*)

18. REASON(S) FOR CONTINUING TREATMENT THIS BILLING PERIOD (Clarify goals and necessity for continued skilled care)

Patient has achieved most STGs but is continuing to make progress toward long-term ambulation goal (current status 500 feet); stair negotiation (currently using STS pattern); and endurance goal (currently 375 feet in 6 minutes).
Patient's limited ROM, pain, and balance impairments are continuing to improve but are limiting functional abilities.
Patient requires skilled PT to focus on remaining LTGs. Skilled PT for 2 weeks. HEP will emphasize ROM, strength and long distance ambulation.

19. SIGNATURE (or name of professional, including prof. designation)	20. DATE	21.
	08/15/2002	[ ] CONTINUE SERVICES OR [X] DC SERVICES

22. FUNCTIONAL LEVEL (at end of billing period - Relate your documentation to functional outcomes and list problems still present)

Patient has achieved all STG and LTGs.
Patient is able to ambulate indoors without an assistive device independently and is able to ambulate 1000 feet with a str cane on all outdoor surfaces independently.
Patient is able to negotiate 24 stairs using s-o-s pattern with 1 rail.
Patient reports pain level to be 1/10 only after extended standing.
AROM (R) Hip Ext/Flex: 0 to 95 degrees
Balance: Proactive and reactive balance has improved, decreasing patient's risk for falls. (BERG BALANCE Score = 50/56)

22. SERVICE DATES	
FROM	THROUGH

FORM HCFA-701 (11-91)

FIGURE 12-4

Sample Medicare HCFA Form 701 completed in a skilled nursing setting.

Attention:
Any Insurance Co.
PO Box 5032
Norwalk, CT 06856-5032

To Whom It May Concern,

I am writing this letter of medical necessity for Jennifer Goodstone for justification for a standing frame for her home. Ms Goodstone is a 68-year-old woman with diagnosis of multiple sclerosis (MS) referred for admission to The County Rehabilitation Hospital 07/23/01 by Dr. Jones. The patient is currently under the care of Dr. Smith. Ms Goodstone was originally diagnosed with relapsing remitting multiple sclerosis in 1995. She has recently been admitted for an MS Exacerbation with a change in the type of MS to progressive MS. Her PMH is significant for myocardial infarction, hypertension, hypercholesterolemia, optic neuritis, RA, CVA, and breast cancer with lumpectomy.

She presents with the following medical/physical status:
- Decreased PROM in bilateral lower extremities with hip extension, hip abduction, and ankle dorsiflexion being most limiting
- Increased bilateral lower extremity tone (spasticity) resulting in decreased ability to perform bowel-bladder routing, transfers, bed mobility, decreased balance in sitting on bed and in wheelchair, and an increase in leg and back pain
- Continent of bowel and bladder with longstanding history or urinary retention
- High risk for osteoporosis of spine and lower extremities secondary to her inability to weight bear through bilateral lower extremities
- Skin is intact but remains at high risk for skin breakdown and pressure sores secondary to inactivity, dependency on wheelchair for mobility and inability to perform effective but independent pressure relief
- Limited functional endurance with significant cardiac history with continued risk for decline secondary to immobility

Currently, Ms Goodstone presents with the following functional mobility status:

TRANSFERS:
- Depression lift transfer wheelchair to/from level mat with supervision
- Sliding board transfer (SBT) wheelchair to/from bed with minimal assistance
- Sit to stand from wheelchair to bed with moderate/maximal assistance
- Stand Pivot Transfer using rolling walker with moderate to maximal assistance to stand and manage right lower extremity during pivot

AMBULATION:
- Patient is currently non-ambulatory. Patient is independent in utilizing a power wheelchair for mobility in hospital environment.

UPRIGHT TOLERANCE:
- Patient tolerates standing table for 30 minutes with appropriate vital signs.

Ms Goodstone is currently receiving multi-disciplinary rehabilitative services at County Rehab of occupational and physical therapy services. In physical therapy, she is receiving daily range of motion, therapeutic exercise, functional mobility training (transfers, bed mobility, standing, etc.), functional endurance training, and wheelchair mobility training. She has been fitted with bilateral leg braces (day and night time) to assist in maintaining lower extremity ROM. In addition to these treatments, she is standing in a standing frame for 30 minutes.

The standing table is utilized to counteract the numerous deleterious effects of immobility on major organ systems in the body: musculoskeletal, renal and urinary tract, skin and underlying tissue, respiratory system, cardiovascular system, and the digestive system. Specifically with Ms Goodstone, the benefits of this treatment are numerous, including: decreased tone/spasticity, decreased pain, improved lower extremity range of motion, improved upright tolerance, improved respiratory status, improvements in cardiovascular status and conditioning, and decreased risk for skin breakdown/pressure sores and osteoporosis. Before this exacerbation, Ms Goodstone was ambulating short household distances with a rolling walker and assistance of her home health aide. With the current diagnosis of progressive MS and her current physical and medical status, she will no longer be able to ambulate. The passive standing allotted by the standing table is essential in providing an effective program for addressing the risks of immobility for this patient in her home.

Thank you for your time and consideration in this matter. Please do not hesitate to contact us directly for any other questions or concerns.

Sincerely,
Joe D. Therapist

FIGURE 12-5

Sample letter to an insurance company requesting specialized equipment. A brief synopsis of patient's status is included, and the specific benefits to the patient are clearly delineated in the second-to-last paragraph.

In reply to: CBA Healthcare Inc.

Attention: Northeast Region Managed Care Division

To Whom It May Concern:

Subject: Request for Additional Physical Therapy Visits for Rupal Patel

Ms. Patel was referred for physical therapy evaluation and treatment 6/15/02, 2 weeks s/p left ankle fracture with ORIF. On initial evaluation this patient presented with pain, edema, decreased ROM and strength, as well as limitations in transfers and ambulatory function. She has received 6/8 authorized physical therapy sessions to date, consisting of moist heat, ultrasound, stretching/strengthening, manual therapy, standing balance, gait training activities, cryotherapy, and patient education in safety precautions and home exercise program activities. This patient has responded well to PT intervention and has achieved the following progress:

Status On Initial Evaluation

- Subjective c/o left ankle pain reported as 8/10 on VAS on all standing/ambulatory activities.
- Figure 8 anthropometric ankle measurements:

  L: 41 cm   R: 35 cm

  AROM:

  PF: 0-10¡   DF: 0¡

  Inversion: 0-7¡   Eversion: 0¡
- Strength:

  PF: 2/5   DF: 2/5

  Supination: 2/5   Pronation: 2/5
- Transfers independently with B axillary crutches using toe-touch WB L LE
- Ambulates independently with B axillary crutches using toe-touch WB L LE for 250 ft on level surfaces and stairs.

Current Status

Patient reports pain has subsided to 4/10 on VAS on left unilateral WB activities.

Figure 8 anthropometric ankle measurements:

L: 37.5 cm   R: 35 cm

- AROM:

  PF: 0-20¡   DF: 0-5¡

  Inversion: 0-15¡   Eversion: 0-7¡
- Strength:

  PF: 3+/5   DF: 4/5

  Supination: 4-/5   Pronation: 4-/5
- Transfers independently with straight cane and WBAT L LE
- Ambulates independently with straight cane WBAT for functional community distances on level surfaces and stairs.

Although significant progress has been achieved, this patient continues to present with the aforementioned impairments/functional limitations limiting her ability to perform her work duties and from participating in recreational activities. This patient requires continued PT treatment 2 x/wk for 4 weeks (8 sessions) as previously described to achieve the following updated PT goals:

- Patient will report decreased pain on all left unilateral WB activities to <2/10 on VAS in 4 weeks/ 8 sessions.
- Patient will display left ankle PF to 30¡, DF to 15¡, supination to 30¡, pronation to 20¡ actively in 4 weeks/8 sessions.
- Patient will display L ankle strength to 4+/5 for PF, DF, supination and pronation in 4 weeks/ 8 sessions.
- Patient will transfer independently without assistive device in 4 weeks/8 sessions.
- Patient will ambulate on level surfaces, ramps (to 15¡ incline), and stairs without assistive device independently in 4 weeks/ 8 sessions.

Thank you for your consideration.

Sincerely,
Jean Smythe, PT

Superior Physical Therapy Group Inc.

FIGURE 12-6

Sample letter to an insurance company requesting approval for additional visits. The letter highlights the patient's quantitative improvements in functional performance, details the skilled intervention that was required to achieve these improvements, and provides evidence to support the benefit of physical therapy and the specific procedures used in this patient population.

PEDIATRICS AND SCHOOL SETTINGS

Early Intervention

Documentation in early intervention, preschool education, and secondary school education involves its own set of documentation standards. Under Part C of the Individuals with Disabilities Education Act (IDEA), infants and toddlers (ages birth to 2 years 11 months) are eligible for early intervention services (physical therapy is considered one type of early intervention service) if they meet the criteria for having a disability. This entails children who (1) are experiencing development delays, as measured by appropriate diagnostic instruments and procedures in any of five developmental domains; (2) have a diagnosed physical or mental condition that has a high probability of resulting in developmental delay; or (3) are at risk of having substantial developmental delays if early intervention services are not provided (McEwen, 2000). Individual states govern the specific eligibility criteria for developmental delay and at-risk children.

PTs are frequently called on to perform evaluations of young children with suspected or known risk for developmental delay, typically in gross or fine motor development. Therapists may perform the evaluation independently, or they may be part of a team of health care professionals who are evaluating a child. In either situation, therapists are required to document the findings from their evaluations. This evaluation serves an important purpose: it provides data on which a decision will be made regarding a child's eligibility for certain early intervention services.

Best practice in early intervention report writing involves several key components. The report should be free of jargon and easily interpreted by individuals outside the medical field (see Chapter 2 for more details on jargon-free note writing). Early intervention evaluations are primarily read by individuals other than health care professionals. They are most often read by individuals from the Department of Health or governing body for the early intervention program, administrators, and most importantly, the child's parents. If medical terminology is required, it should be defined whenever possible.

Evaluations should focus not only on the problems or things that the child cannot do, but rather on what he or she is able to do. Deficiencies can, and should, be highlighted in the report, but the overall tone of the evaluation should be centered on the child's abilities at the present time.

Although the criteria for eligibility vary among states, most criteria are based on scores from standardized tests (although other information, including informed clinical opinion, is often considered). Use of standardized testing whenever possible is critical for therapists who perform early intervention evaluations; the results of the standardized tests should be documented in the evaluation report. When a standardized test, such as the Peabody Developmental Motor Scales-edition 2 (PDMS-2) (Folio and Fewell, 2000), is used as a measure of gross motor function in young children, the evaluation report should not focus solely on the results of the test and the child's performance on specific items. The PDMS, or any other test, only provides representative test items to evaluate children and determine their motor score compared with other children their age. It does not presume to evaluate every area of gross motor function. Thus therapists must use clinical judgment to determine other areas of motor functioning and impairments to test. Documentation therefore should reflect a well-rounded assessment of a child's disability, or potential disability, the functional abilities and limitations (typically motor skills and self-care skills), and any related impairments.

The PDMS-2 and the motor scale of the Bayley Scales of Infant Development-II (Bayley, 2001) are two of the most commonly used discriminative measures in early intervention. Discriminative measures "distinguish between children who have and do not have a particular characteristic" (McEwen, 2000). Such measures are necessary in early intervention to distinguish between children who are developing typically and those who have delays in development. Both the PDMS and the Bayley scales are norm-referenced, which provides for age-based comparisons. Thus a child receives a score, typically a mean and a standard deviation (SD), or a Z score, which provides information about how far from the mean a child's skills are. Many states have explicit eligibility criteria stated in terms of number of standard deviations from the mean (e.g., children who fall at or below 2 SD from the mean in one or more developmental domains qualify for services) or percentiles (e.g., children who fall below the 5th percentile.

In some cases, standardized testing is not appropriate for a specific child. He or she may not be able to follow directions to perform a specific test, or no test may be developed to measure the child's specific problems. In these cases, informed clinical opinion is warranted. Sometimes, when children have severe motor impairments, the norms developed for a specific test may no longer be valid. Therapists therefore must provide compelling documentation to explain the nature of the child's problem and why and how it does or may result in delayed development.

Additional information on these concepts and best practice guidelines for conducting and documenting early intervention evaluation reports can be found in the (Towle and O'Hara, 1995). Figure 12-7 provides a checklist for evaluation reports from this workbook to ensure that key components are appropriately addressed.

Individual family service plans (IFSPs) are required documentation for any child receiving early intervention services. This plan serves as the "contract" between the state governing agency and the family to outline the goals of early intervention for a child (McEwen, 2000). PTs are typically required to document a summary of a child's gross motor skills and goals for their continued development. These goals must be written in collaboration with the family and thus should be clearly written with specific measurable activities and time frames. IDEA mandates a review of the IFSP every 6 months. A sample IFSP summary and goals is shown in Figure 12-8.

School-Based Intervention

Older children (typically ages 3 to 21 years, depending on state policy) "are eligible for special education and related services (e.g., physical therapy) if they meet the eligibility criteria for one of the 13 categories of disabilities specified under IDEA, and require special education and related services because of the disability" (McEwen, 2000, p. 12). Although early intervention services are typically provided in the child's home, children with disabilities who are older than age 3 receive services in a school setting. For these children, individualized education plans (IEPs) are developed as mandated under Part B of IDEA. These education plans are multidisciplinary and are completed by the personnel involved with the child's education. IEPs are designed differently by each state. In most states, therapists are required to write a summary of a child's physical functioning and health status as it affects his or her performance in the school setting and document goals for the upcoming year. IDEA mandates review of the IEP on a yearly basis. Thus therapists, educators, and other providers must write a new IEP with new goals for the upcoming year.

Figure 12-9 provides an example of a yearly IEP summary and goals related to a child's physical growth and development. Therapists are typically involved in writing components of the IEP that are related to the specific services they are providing. Arguably, the most important component of the IEP is the goals. The annual goals provide the foundation for the type of activities that should be addressed during the upcoming year. According to McEwen (2000), annual goals should "be functional, discipline-free, chronologically age-appropriate, and meaningful to the students and the students' family. They should also include activities that the student can perform frequently and they should address both the present and the future needs of the student." (p. 54). Goal writing on the IEP is meant to address specific goals related to functioning in the school. Therefore writing strictly impairment-related goals in this setting is not meaningful. Goals are read by parents and school personnel, who are often not familiar with medical terminology. Therapists should avoid jargon and define terms when necessary (also see Chapter 2 for more on avoiding jargon).

Functional outcomes documentation is very important in the school setting. The purpose of a PT's evaluation and intervention within the school setting is to help the child function better in the school (i.e., in the lunchroom, classroom, playground, etc.). In addition to writing summary information and goals on the IEP, therapists may complete a full evaluation. The focus of this documentation should be on how limitations in physical functioning and gross motor skills affect the child's ability to function in the school setting. This could relate to a child's ability to move within a classroom or between classrooms, to participate in gym class or on the playground, to climb stairs in the school, to get on and off the bus, or to participate in self-care skills such as dressing and toileting. The School Function Assessment (Coster et al., 1998) provides a standardized format for therapists to evaluate such limitations.

SUMMARY

- This chapter provides an overview of various kinds of specialized documentation in physical therapy, including discharge notes, patient education materials, Medicare forms and pediatric-specific documentation (IFSPs and IEPs).

- All forms of patient documentation should be concise, free of jargon, and focus on the important aspects related to the patient's plan of care and improving the functional outcomes.

- Although formats and requirements (particularly for Medicare) change frequently, the principles related to functional outcomes approach provide a consistent framework for all types of documentation.

QUALITY IMPROVEMENT INVENTORY
Early Intervention Reports

Name of Child:_____ MR#:_____

Date of Evaluation:_____

Type of Evaluation: EI   Family Program   Other:_____

Clinicians:_____

_____

Rater:_____

	not at all	somewhat	very much
1. Clearly states reason for referral	1	2	3
2. Has form and/or organization	1	2	3
3. Includes neutral observation of child	1	2	3
4. Testing conditions are noted	1	2	3
5. Explains the instruments or evaluation approaches being used	1	2	3
6. Results are complete	1	2	3
7. Explains the meaning of results	1	2	3
8. Results are interpreted in light of referral question	1	2	3
9. Results include parent input or report	1	2	3
10. Results are explained without jargon or jargon is defined	1	2	3
11. Conclusions and recommendations emerge logically	1	2	3
12. Recommendations are detailed enough	1	2	3
13. Provides motivation to follow recommendations	1	2	3
14. Shows how problems came about	1	2	3
15. Includes strengths	1	2	3
16. Is strength-oriented	1	2	3
17. Is free of typos, grammatical, spelling errors	1	2	3
18. Summary reiterates and addresses referral questions	1	2	3
19. Enjoyable to read	1	2	3
20. Summary/recommendations reflect parent reaction to feedback	1	2	3

Other comments:_____

_____

_____

_____

Jargon not defined in text:_____

_____

_____

_____

FIGURE 12-7

Quality Improvement Inventory outlines 20 key components to appropriate documentation for Early Intervention reports. Such a form can be used for peer-review or as part of ongoing quality improvement.

Courtesy A. Farrell, PhD.

INDIVIDUALIZED FAMILY SERVICE PLAN

Summary of Child's Present Abilities, Strengths, and Needs

Maddie L. is a very content 13-month-old baby, who enjoys sitting and standing activities. She plays independently in ring, sitting on the floor (with knees to either side and feet together). She demonstrates the ability to turn her trunk while sitting with no difficulty. She stands at the couch when placed there. She is not cruising (walking along the furniture) to the left or right at this time. She will walk with hands held or behind a push toy. When she walks, she keeps the left side of her pelvis retracted (pulled back), and her left hip and leg externally rotated (turned out to the side) on approximately 50% of the steps.

Maddie is a mobile child. She scoots on her behind, using her left arm and right leg as her main points of push off. She keeps her left leg fully extended in front of her while scooting around. She maintains her right arm in her lap while moving around. If she is placed in quadruped position (hands and knees in contact with the floor) she is able to reciprocally crawl, although the movement is stiff looking, with a wide base of support at the knees. She is unable to transition out of this quadruped position into sitting without assistance.

Transitions appear to be the biggest area of difficulty for Maddie. She is able to play in prone (on her belly), fully extending her arms and weight shifting but is unable to roll off her belly and onto her back and vice versa. She is able to ring sit and play independently, but is unable to get herself into, or out of sitting without assistance. She is able to stand at the couch, or walk behind a push toy, but is unable to pull herself into the standing position. Without mastering these essential transitions, Maddie is now behind where she should be developmentally.

In terms of physical impairments, Maddie has no passive or active range of motion limitations discovered during physical examination. She demonstrates some weakness in her trunk and shoulder muscle, as evidenced by limitations in certain transitional skills and ability to fully bear weight through her hands. She did not demonstrate any atypical reflexes.

According to the Peabody Developmental Scales (mean = 10, SD = 3), Maddie achieved a raw score of 4 on the locomotion subtest and 5 on the stationary subtest. This indicates that Maddie fell approx. 2 SD below the mean in gross motor skills. This score places Maddie at <1 percentile rank. This is a significant delay and she would benefit from direct early intervention services. These services should be aimed at helping her to improve her gross motor skills to within age-appropriate parameters.

OBJECTIVES
1. Maddie will roll supine to prone and back independently (1 month)
2. Maddie will transition from a supine position, rolling to her side and coming to sit independently 4/5 times (1 month)
3. Maddie will independently transition from ring sit to quadruped and back 4/5 times (2 months)
4. Maddie will pull to stand at the couch and cruise independently for a toy placed 5 feet away (2 months)
5. Maddie will transition to stand without support and will stand independently for 10 seconds (4 months)
6. Maddie will walk across the family room with supervision (6 months)

FIGURE 12-8

Component of an Individualized Family Service Plan (IFSP): summary and objectives related to a child's motor development.

Student _*Phil O'Connor*_

ANNUAL GOALS AND SHORT-TERM OBJECTIVES

There will be __*3*__ reports of progress per year.

ANNUAL GOAL: *Phil will negotiate open environments (playground, classroom, hallway) within or around the school community with supervision only, during all transitions throughout the school day.*	PROGRESS:	1st	2nd	3rd
	Methods of Measurement			
	Report of Progress			
	Progress Toward Annual Goal			
	Reasons for not Meeting Annual Goal			

SHORT-TERM OBJECTIVES:

1. Phil will utilize his walker for outside ambulation activities given only distant supervision and including all terrains (ramp, curb, sidewalk, pavement). 5/5 trials per week

2. Phil will ambulate during the school day within the school environment, without utilizing his posterior walker, for all activities/transitions, given distant supervision. 5/5 days

ANNUAL GOAL: *Phil will negotiate 2 flights of stairs given distant supervision by classroom staff and utilizing 1 rail hold with a step over step pattern, 3/3 trials per day.*	PROGRESS:	1st	2nd	3rd
	Methods of Measurement			
	Report of Progress			
	Progress Toward Annual Goal			
	Reasons for not Meeting Annual Goal			

SHORT-TERM OBJECTIVES:

1. Phil will ascend/descend 1 flight of stairs given intermittent tactile and verbal cues 2/2 trials, utilizing 1 rail hold and step over step pattern.

2. Phil will ascend/descend 1 flight of stairs utilizing 1 rail hold and step over step pattern with close supervision only, 3/3 trials

EXPLANATION OF CODING SYSTEM

METHODS OF MEASUREMENT

1. Teacher Made Materials
2. Standardized Tests
3. Class Activities
4. Portfolio(s)
5. Teacher/Provider Observations_____

6. Performance Assessment Task
7. Check Lists
8. Verbal Explanation
9. Other (Specify)_____

REPORT OF PROGRESS

1. Not applicable during this grading period
2. No progress made
3. Little progress made
4. Progress made; goal not yet met
5. Goal met

PROGRESS TOWARD GOAL

A. Anticipate meeting goal
B. Do not anticipate meeting goal (Note reason)
C. Goal met

REASONS FOR NOT MEETING GOAL

1. More time needed
2. Excessive absence or lateness
3. Assignments not completed
4. Other (specify) _____

FIGURE 12-9

Sample Individualized Education Plan (IEP) summary and goals for a child receiving physical therapy in a public school. The goals of the IEP are related to the child's functioning within the school setting and are objective and measurable.

Continued

Student _____ *Phil O'Connor* _____

HEALTH AND PHYSICAL DEVELOPMENT

PRESENT HEALTH STATUS AND PHYSICAL DEVELOPMENT:

Phil has had a difficult and lengthy recovery from multiple surgeries to his legs in October (tendon releases to gastrocs & hamstrings). He continues to require follow-up care and is now followed by Dr. Jones at Community Hospital. Phil typically has excellent attendance and exhibits good health and development. He is followed by a nephrologist once a year.

MEDICAL/HEALTH CARE NEEDS

During the school day, the student requires:

Oral medication   ☐ Yes ☑ No
(If yes, functionally describe the condition for which medication is required.)

_____

Treatment(s) or other health procedure(s)   ☐ Yes ☑ No
(If yes, functionally describe the condition for which treatment(s) or procedure(s) are required.)

_____

Health as a related service   ☐ Yes ☑ No
(If yes, specify in related service recommendations.)

_____

PHYSICAL NEEDS

The student   ☑ does ☐ does not have mobility limitations.
(If yes, functionally describe the limitation(s).)

requires walker for outdoor terrain.
_____

The student requires:

Accessible program   ☑ Yes ☐ No

Adaptive physical education   ☑ Yes ☐ No

Assistive technology device(s) ☐ Yes ☑ No

Assistive technology service(s) ☐ Yes ☑ No
(If assistive technology device(s) or service(s) are required, specify in management needs.)

HEALTH/PHYSICAL MANAGEMENT NEEDS
(Environmental modifications, human/material resources or specialized equipment)

Phil utilizes a posterior walker for outdoor ambulation. He is currently awaiting a manual wheelchair for trips of longer durations. He will utilize an orthosis for his right foot and has a lift in his left shoe. Phil has a shunt in place without problems in recent history and utilizes eyeglasses throughout the day.

FIGURE 12-9—cont'd

CHAPTER 13

Automating Physical Therapy Documentation

JANET HERBOLD

LEARNING OBJECTIVES

After reading this chapter and completing the exercises, the reader will be able to:

1. Identify the benefits of an automated documentation system.
2. Understand the key considerations when determining the appropriate use for an automated system.
3. Describe the process of effectively selecting and implementing an automated computerized clinical documentation system.

Traditional physical therapy documentation has been done using a pen and paper method. Some clinics and institutions use completely narrative notes, whereas others have migrated to preprinted forms. Preprinted forms are in effect a way in which physical therapy documentation has become more automated over the past few decades. As the twenty-first century progresses, the computer will have a significant impact on physical therapy practice, most significantly documentation. Some institutions already have made the transition to various forms of computerized documentation. This chapter highlights the pros and cons of using computerized documentation and some considerations for choosing a package that best meets the needs of an institution.

Almost any therapist can attest to the inherent drawbacks to the pen and paper method of documentation. The first is the legibility of the notes. Illegibly handwritten notes can lead to denied payment and errors in clinical practice. The use of abbreviations is another significant factor inherent in handwritten notes. Without an established standard list of abbreviations, it is difficult for many outside the physical therapy profession to interpret notes written in physical therapy jargon or loaded with abbreviations (see Chapter 2). Redundancy

of medical and demographic information is another disadvantage to pen and paper notes. Therapists frequently copy information written by another health care professional into their own notes. Such facts as the patient's diagnosis, date of birth, past medical history, and medications are frequently manually rewritten onto therapy documentation (see Chapter 4). In addition, as the completion of regulatory forms such as Inpatient Rehabilitation Facility—Patient Assessment Instrument (IRF-PAI), Minimum Data Set-Resource Utilization Groups (MDS-RUGS), and Outcome and Assessment and Information Set (OASIS) become necessary for reimbursement and payment, therapists, nurses, physicians, and social workers must document in the medical record and on the reimbursement form. Both of these practices result in redundancy and duplication of documentation at a time in health care when efficiency of clinical practice and staff productivity are being scrutinized. Finally, the pen and paper method does not allow for easy data retrieval for clinical research or outcomes analysis. It has become increasingly important to demonstrate treatment effectiveness through clinical research. Pen and paper notation is very difficult, and manual review and analysis of notes in charts to determine treatment effectiveness is time consuming. In many cases the variation in note writing style and terminology make it impossible to extract comparative data from handwritten notes from different clinicians even for the same type of patient.

During an age of maximizing productivity, accessing clinical data to report outcomes, and reduced length of stay in patient days, therapists seek creative ways to streamline documentation in a method that reduces redundancy and error and facilitates data retrieval. As a result, some facilities have purchased or developed computerized therapy records.

The purpose of an automated clinical documentation system is to create an environment that supports and facilitates a well-developed evaluation or note. A well-written note, whether handwritten or computer-driven, should help the clinician identify clearly the functional problems facing the patient and develop an appropriate plan of care. The process of documentation should assist with the creation of functionally relevant goals and a corresponding treatment plan. The decision to create or use a computerized system for physical therapy documentation for any or all aspects of the medical record can lead to exciting and thought-provoking discussions. Whether the practice is a freestanding outpatient facility or a large department with a multilayered continuum, many employees and departments must be included in the discussion to move toward an integrated approach to documentation and billing. Some key players in this initial decision-making process include the hospital's or facility's director/chief executive officer (CEO)/chief operating officer (COO); the financial departments or chief financial officer (CFO); information services (IS); the medical and nursing staff; rehabilitation services of physical therapy, occupational therapy, speech therapy, and recreational therapy; social work/case management, and financial services (billing and collection). Each member of the team brings unique perspective regarding the benefits, drawbacks, and issues that should be considered through the proposed automated solution.

SYSTEM BENEFITS

Standardization of Data Elements and Charting Practices

A computerized system can create a standard data collection tool format for the evaluation, daily charting sessions, reevaluations, and discharge evaluations. Therapists can use a variety of devices to access and chart in the electronic medical recording. Devices such as laptop computers and hand-held devices allow clinicians to document during the patient evaluation and treatment with the patient present. This is referred to as point-of-care (PDC)

documentation. The therapist naturally becomes faster and more efficient as a note writer simply through repetition and practice. In addition, training of new or rotating staff members is easier and more consistent throughout the organization. Computerized documentation allows consistent collection of data elements for a specific patient type in which the same information can be captured in the same order for all patients. This standardization helps those reading the documentation as they become familiar with the format and are able to locate pertinent information quickly and easily. Furthermore, specific terminology can be written into the computer programs to provide consistency among therapists, as well as reduce the use of abbreviations.

Figure 13-1 illustrates these features in a software program (MediServe Information System, Tempe, Ariz) with templates designed by a team of rehabilitation professionals (Burke Rehabilitation Hospital, White Plains, NY). In this example the Impression/Assessment is coded to include key components such as summarizing and drawing relationships between the patient's impairments, functional limitations, and disability (to develop the physical therapy diagnosis). All possible options for each of these components are listed as options in a pull-down menu (in this example, Life Role Participation). By using such a format, therapists are prompted to provide critical information so that it will always be included in their documentation. Furthermore, the design of the template is structured so that the terminology is consistent with current practice, and importantly, the *Guide to Physical Therapist Practice*.

Standardized assessment tools also can be easily incorporated into evaluations, assessments, and daily notes and thus be a part of the therapist's documentation system. Figure 13-2 illustrates how a standardized test, such as the 6-minute walk test, can be easily incorporated into computerized documentation. This allows outcomes data collection and retrieval as a by-product of charting instead of a separate and lengthy chart review process.

Elimination of Redundancy and Reduction of Errors

Most hospitals and facilities already have computerized registration, financial services, and scheduling systems, or a combination of these three components, in which basic patient demographic information is entered and stored. Through the use of interface technology and connectivity, patient demographic and clinical data can be directly fed into a computerized documentation system by simply selecting the patient and verifying an account or medical record number. This practice of sharing information between systems significantly reduces the documentation time normally required to rewrite that necessary information onto a paper form. In addition,

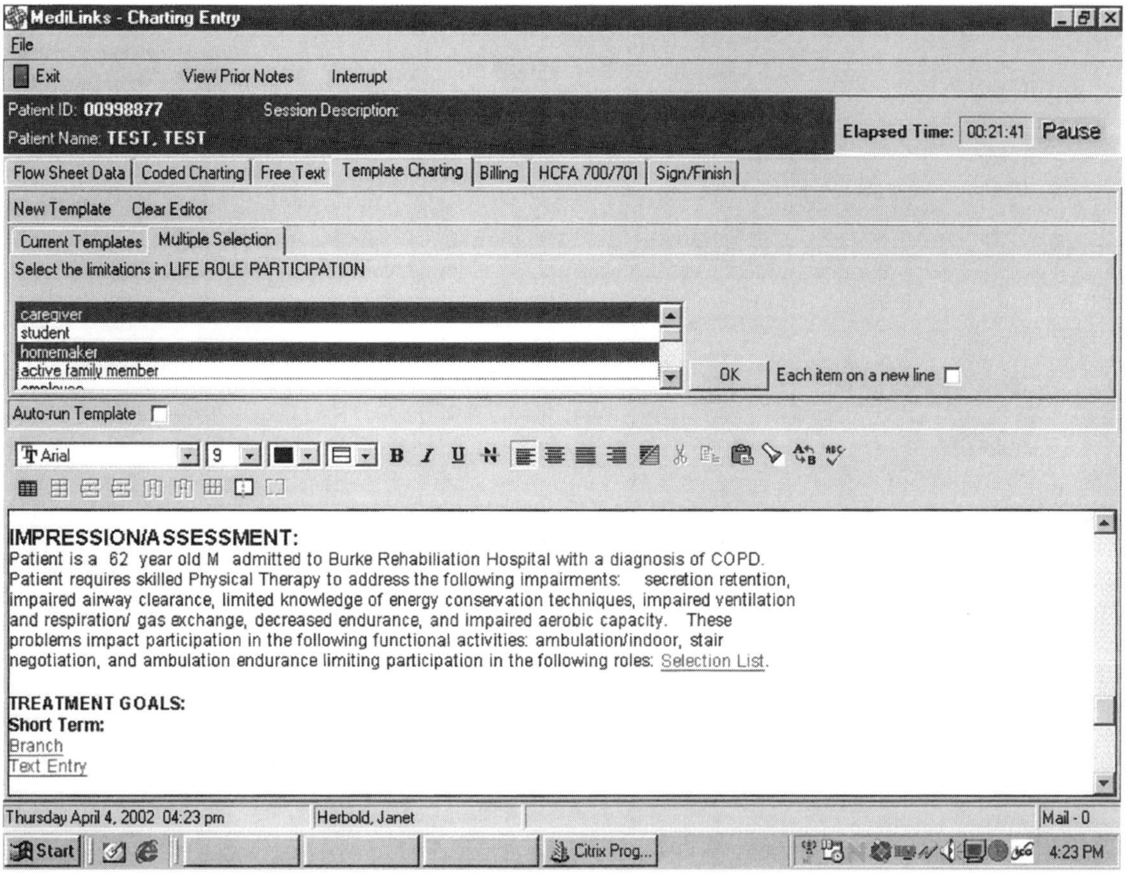

FIGURE 13-1

Computerized documentation template for the Assessment section of an initial evaluation. Selection lists are available at various points throughout the documentation. This figure illustrates the output of selection lists of impairments and functional limitations.

it also reduces the human error that can be associated with such transcription practices.

Just as information can be received *into* an electronic documentation system, it also can be forwarded *out* to another system. This is the case with the interface into a billing or data collection system. Such an interface allows billing/charging elements to be forwarded or interfaced into the financial system, again reducing potential billing error and billing/charting discrepancies by eliminating an extra step in the documentation and billing practices. Current reimbursement regulations require a perfect match between items billed and treatment rendered. Inconsistencies in documentation and billing could result in reimbursement denials. The practice of "marrying" documentation with billing helps to alleviate those issues reducing potential denials.

Accessibility of Data in "Real Time"

In many facilities an inherent time delay occurs between when and where the notes are documented and when

they are accessible in the medical record. Therapy notes are frequently written and maintained in a clinic and later transferred into the medical record. Not having access to clinical data close to the time that it is written can greatly reduce the hospital's efficiency and facilitation of the continuum of care within a facility, as well as across networked or other facility sites. Use of an automated clinical documentation system allows easy accessibility of clinical information both at remote locations from where services have been provided and immediately after documentation of the encounter. Access to therapy notes by physicians, nursing staff, social workers, and case managers allows the rehabilitation process to be continued and reported over the full 24-hour a day period. Physicians can discuss current functional status with their patients, family members, and caregivers at any time during the patient's stay. The availability of clinical data can help the physician make medical choices and discuss discharge planning options with confidence in a timely manner. The nursing staff can promote and carry through the rehabilitation process 24 hours a day, 7 days per week by having access to the

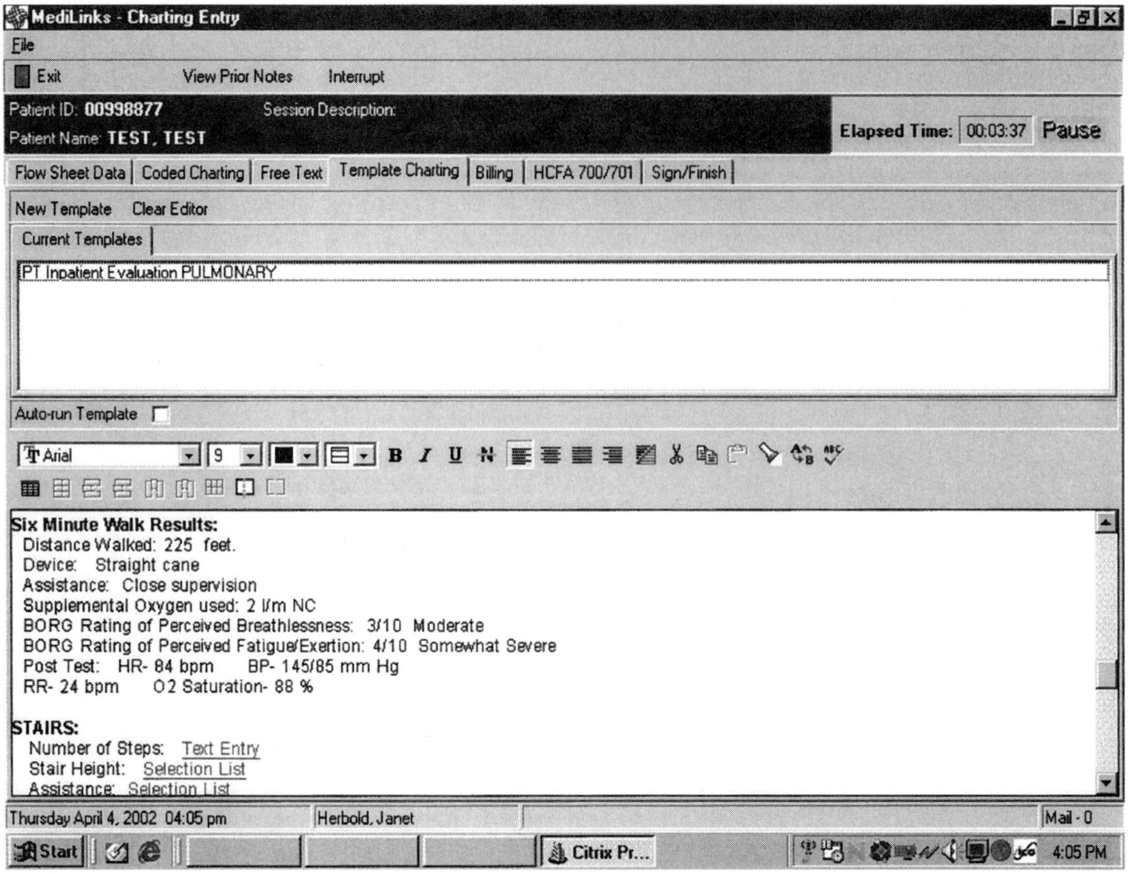

FIGURE 13-2

Illustration of how computerized documentation can use standardized assessment tools (e.g., 6-minute walk) into the body of a charting template. This provides a means of quickly and easily documenting standard information for a specific patient population.

patient's most recent physical status. Social workers and case managers can easily access and send updated functional status reports to insurance companies, external case managers, and other necessary medical continuum levels to facilitate communication regarding patient status, transfer, and discharge process. The benefits of an automated environment help to instill confidence in the medical facility and promote efficiency in the care of the patient.

In addition to sending and receiving information within a facility, connectivity across different hospitals or sites promotes a clinically integrated delivery system. Allowing access to clinical care data across the continuum of patient services, such as from an acute care hospital to a rehabilitation center or an outpatient environment, promotes continued medical and rehabilitation care without interruption. Availability of clinical data throughout the rehabilitation continuum ultimately leads to improved functional outcome, better patient satisfac-

tion, and more camaraderie among caregivers and personnel. As patients move from one site or facility to another, the evaluation process of "getting to know" the patient can be reduced through availability of the most recent functional status and rehabilitation report. Because patients can continue to progress in their rehabilitation process, outcomes and patient satisfaction can be improved. In addition, the communication of patient information from one therapist to another helps to facilitate professional interaction and development of best practice.

Cost Efficiency

The current age in health care mandates demonstration of treatment effectiveness and efficiency of services. For this reason and because of the need to do so without added cost to the system, monitoring of

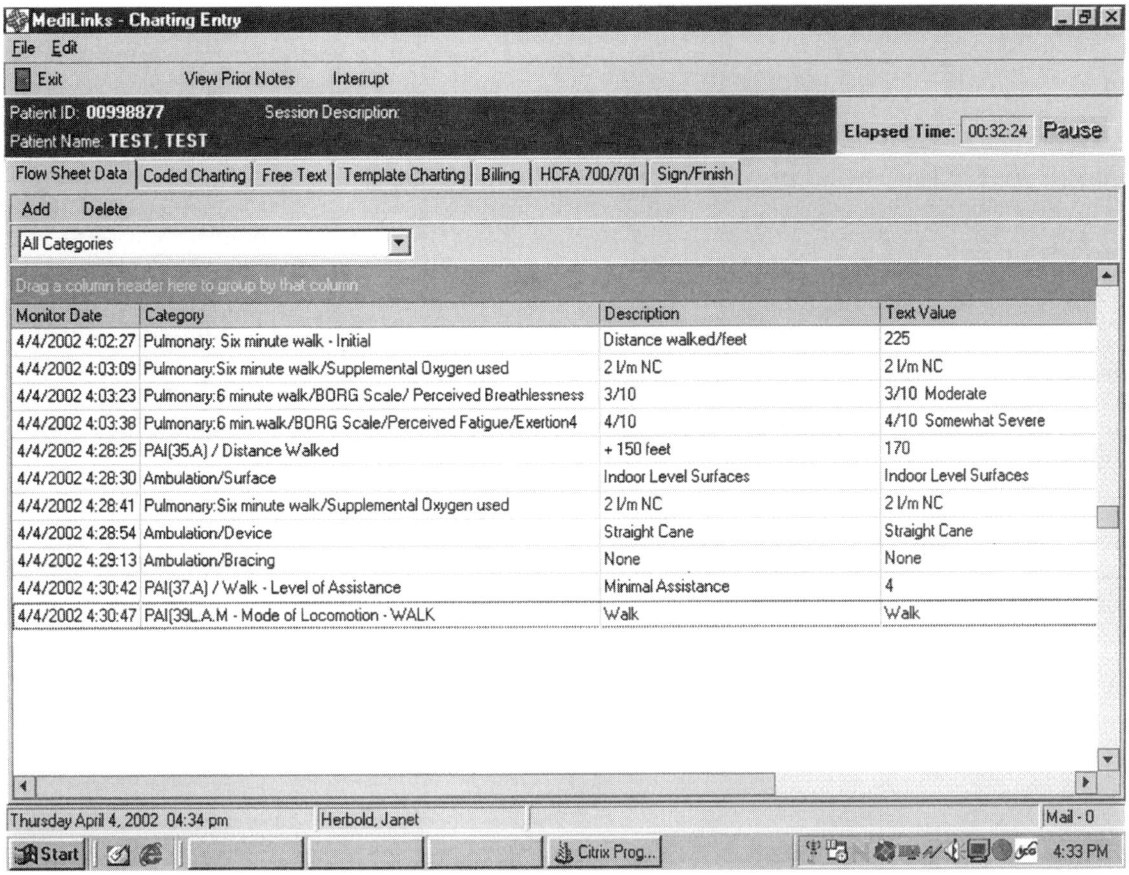

FIGURE 13-3

Specific tests and measures gleaned from an initial evaluation report. Computerized documentation can capture important charting elements and use them in an outcome report based on patient type.

clinical data must necessarily be incorporated as a component of documentation and charting. The availability of data in a computerized form can allow analysis of clinical outcomes and cost of services. The use of computer analysis simplifies demonstration of efficiency and effectiveness to patients, third-party payers, accrediting bodies, stakeholders, and therapists themselves.

Functional Outcomes Assessment

Computerized documentation allows outcome data collection elements to be charted during routine documentation and simultaneously entered into its own system. Without computerized documentation, outcomes measures, such as the functional independent measures (FIM) and the Minimum Data Set–Resource Utilization Groups (MDS-RUGS) items, must be documented separately in the therapy notes and the standardized forms. Automated documentation systems allow the information to be imbedded in a documentation template and transferred to a freestanding electronic documentation such as an MDS or FIM report. Figure 13-3 provides an example of various tests and outcomes measures that can be gleaned from chart documentation for a patient with a pulmonary condition. Such direct routing of clinical information into regulatory reporting systems for outcome analysis demonstrates a more efficient system with fewer redundancies and reduced errors.

SYSTEM CONSIDERATIONS

The primary drawbacks to the use of an automated documentation system include the initial financial investment, development time, and staff training. An automated electronic rehabilitation system could cost as much as $1 million for the system itself. Additional expenses include the time for staff development of the software. Some software systems provide "canned" documentation tools with the ability to modify them, whereas others allow the flexibility for total customization but thus require additional time and resources for development. Experience suggests that it will take up to a year to fully develop charting templates or modify canned templates for facility use.

Finally, time and resources must be allocated for staff training for the basic computer level and specific application training. A well-developed training tool should include basic computer training for skills such as opening and closing applications; cutting, copying, and pasting functions; mouse skills; highlighting and deleting text; and basic typing skills. Once the staff is comfortable with basic word-processing functions, application training should begin approximately 2 weeks before the implementation or "go-live" date. Application training should incorporate thorough understanding and functionality of the software, practice with actual charting templates that the specific user may use, and knowledge of how to view other notes, print files, and access clinically relevant patient demographic information. Such application training probably requires between 3 and 4 hours. After the go-live date the training becomes part of the ongoing maintenance of the application for future users because of staff turnover. Training is only one of the many ongoing tasks involved in system maintenance. Others include entering new users in the practitioner file, updating the charge master as changes to billing and reimbursement are identified, and modifying existing documentation templates as changes in regulatory requirements become known.

PROCESS

This section outlines the process that a facility should follow to effectively select and implement an automated computerized documentation system.

Development of a Request for Proposal

Before the vendor interview and selection process, the hospital, rehabilitation institution, or outpatient facility must create a list of all the functions that the institution requires from its automated documentation solution. Each item or functional aspect should be written and included in a document that is submitted and answered by each prospective vendor. It will be beneficial to involve the therapist or end-users in this process, including those with computer backgrounds, as well as

novice computer users. The early involvement of clinical staff in the process will help promote the transition from paper notes to computerized documentation and prevent leaving out a key system element. The request for proposal (RFP) document must be complete because it will become the essence of the vendor/site contract.

During vendor selection the RFP should be used as a checklist to ensure complete functionality of a proposed system based on the identified needs of the site or institution. The vendors must return this document identifying the availability of each item requested. The vendor should indicate whether the item is presently available, will be available soon, will be available in the future in a later release, or is not available in the proposed system.

Vendor Selection

Choice of a vendor is a critical decision in the overall process leading to automation. The institution and the vendor will become partners in a long-term relationship. Both parties must be comfortable with one another and possess a mutual respect. During the vendor selection process, institutions should choose a vendor whose system best matches the long-term plans and needs of the institution. Purchase of a fully comprehensive electronic medical record keeping system is not necessary if the institution does not plan to use all of its functions. Institutions should consider small-niche vendors that specialize in the institution's unique area of expertise in rehabilitation and those systems with total functionality and the ability to integrate throughout a hospital network. A thoroughly prepared RFP will assist the institution and the vendor in knowing the institution's specific needs and the vendor's ability to accomplish them.

Creating a Timeline

Before the automation project is launched, planning and identification of all of the critical elements in the project and the responsible parties is critical. This can be accomplished with a timeline and a responsibility list. Planning the project in this manner will assist the institution in ensuring that all necessary tasks have been identified. Maintenance of this document can be time consuming, but identification of the critical events in the project and completion in the proper sequence are important factors. Similar to building a house, the process begins with the vendor (contractor) selection and the RFP (architect's plans) and proceeds to the template development (building phase), ending with implementation and final acceptance (final inspection and moving in). As with any building project, realistic timeframes should be given, and extra time must be incorporated for unexpected delays.

Design/Validation Team

Depending on the system selected the design/validation team works on developing the charting or note writing templates to be used in the system. The staff selected for this role should be experienced and well versed in the reimbursement practices and financial constraints of the institution.

The goal of this team is to develop standard, consistent formats and data elements with corresponding outcome monitoring tools. Templates can differ between diagnostic categories to capture unique clinically significant assessment data, but a standard format should be used for all charting types. This will assist those completing and reading the templates to maintain a consistent and predictable flow and order. Whenever possible, selection lists and discrete text data elements should be used as charting prompts for data entry and data collection to allow retrieval of the data for later analysis. Narrative or text answers cannot be analyzed and used for comparative analysis. In addition, abbreviations should be kept to a minimum. The speed benefits of using abbreviations on manual charting practices do not exist with computerized documents and will detract from the readability of the notes.

Standardized assessment tools should be incorporated into the templates. This feature will facilitate research and outcome studies as a by-product of daily note writing. In addition, documentation templates should contain those standard elements needed to comply with the facility's outcome or reimbursement tools such as the FIMware (property of University of Buffalo Foundation Activities, Inc.) and IRF–PAI documents (Figure 13-4). These standard elements should be interfaced directly into the unique system to maintain efficiency and reduce redundancy and potential error.

Training Team

The key to a successful computerized implementation is in the training. A careful hands-on training workshop is necessary before implementation. The training should meet the needs of novice and experienced computer users. It will need to incorporate basic computer skills and mouse training, as well as the actual software training. Handouts and reference material, as well as a supervised practice lab, will further enhance the education and confidence level of the new end-user. Training will become an ongoing process as a result of staff turnover and software system upgrades.

Technical Resources and Support Team   The resources brought forth by the information services department are critical. Their expertise will be involved in determining the best technologic solution possible for operation and connectivity needs based on financial resources, modern technology, and building structure.

Hardware selection will be an important consideration. There are many hardware options available to support system use and encourage POC documentation. Mounted laptops on rolling carts are frequently used in one or two room clinics and those areas requiring constant network connections; hand-held devices that require uploading and downloading software are used in facilities where constant connection is not possible and in facilities with multiple sites and home care settings. Personal Digital Assistants (PDAs) allow full connection and maintain adequate mobility for the hospital, as well as an off-site environment. The technologic solution selected will depend on the need for portability, the available connections, the site locations where the system will be used, and financial resources.

Cost Effectiveness

There is little available in the literature supporting the financial return on investment (ROI) with computer documentation systems because of limited experience and time. Some of the potential areas in which computerized documentation could provide cost savings include secretarial support, dictation, and man-power time. Computerized documentation systems reduce redundancy by combining billing and regulatory data with clinical documentation. Furthermore, computerized documentation can reduce denial rates by prompting all therapists to include required data. The appeals process for reimbursement denials is very costly and time consuming for therapists and administrative staff.

Data from one facility* that recently changed to computerized documentation suggests that the therapist may be more satisfied with various components of an automated documentation system vs. a pen-and-paper method. Of the PT staff surveyed 85% stated that they preferred computerized documentation over pen and paper, 100% of the staff believed that patient documentation by other professionals was more accessible in an automated documentation system than accessing information via the chart, and 84% stated that computerized documentation was more efficient. These data suggest that therapists who use computerized documentation systems may have higher job satisfaction, which may result in better staffing retention.

---

*Data collected at Burke Rehabilitation Hospital, White Plains, New York.

Identification Information

1. Facility Information

   A. Facility Name

   Burke Rehabilitation Hospital

   B. Facility Medicare Provider Number

2. Patient Medicare Number

3. Patient Medicaid Number

4. Patient First Name

5. Patient Last Name

6. Birth Date   07/07/1929
                                                 MM/DD/YYYY

7. Social Security Number   000000001

8. Gender (1- Male; 2- Female)   1

9. Race/Ethnicity (Check all that apply)

   American Indian or Alaska Native   A
   Asian   B
   Black or African American   C
   Hispanic or Latino   D
   Native Hawaiian or Other Pacific Islander E
   White   F

10. Marital Status   02

    1 - Never Married; 2- Married; 3 - Widowed;
    4 - Separated; 5 - Divorced

11. Zip Code of Patient's Pre-Hospital Residence: 10605

Admission Information*

12. Admission Date   09/12/2002
                                       (MM/DD/YYYY)

13. Assessment Reference Date   09/14/2002
                                       (MM/DD/YYYY)

14. Admission Class   01
    (1- Initial Rehab; 2 - Evaluation; 3 - Readmission; 4 - Unplanned
    Discharge; 5 - Continuing Rehabilitation

15. Admit From   07
    (01 - Home; 02 - Board & Care; 03 - Transitional Living; 04 -
    Intermediate Care; 05 - Skilled Nursing Facility; 06 - Acute Unit of
    Own Facility; 07 - Acute Unit of Another Facility; 08 - Chronic
    Hospital; 09 - Rehabilitation Facility; 10 - Other; 12 - Alternate Level
    of Care Unit; 13 - Subacute Setting; 14 - Assisted Living Residence)

16. Pre Hospital Living Setting   01
    (Use codes from item 15 above)

17. Pre-Hospital Living With   02
    (Code only if item 16 is 01 - Home; Score using 1 - Alone; 2
    - Family/Relatives; 3 - Friends; 4 - Attendant; 5 - Other)

18. Pre-Hospital Vocational Category   06
    (1 - Employed; 2 - Sheltered; 3 - Student; 4 -
    Homemaker; 5 - Not Working; 6 - Retired for Age; 7 -
    Retired for Disability

19. Pre-Hospital Vocational Effort
    (Code only if item 18 is coded 1 - 4; Score using 1 - Full
    time; 2 - Part time; 3 - Adjusted Workload)

Payer Information

20. Payment Source

    A. Primary Source

    B. Secondary Source

    (Score using 01 - Blue Cross; 02 - Medicare non-MCO; 03 - Medicaid
    non-MCO; 04 - Commercial Insurance; 05 - MCO HMO; 06 - Workers
    Compensation; 07 - Crippled Children's Service; 08 - Developmental
    Disabilities Service; 09 - State Vocational Rehabilitation; 10 - Private
    Pay; 11 - Employee Courtesy; 12 - Unreimbursed; 13 - CHAMPUS; 14 -
    Other; 15 - None; 16 - No Fault auto insurance; 51 - Medicare MCO; 52
    - Medicaid MCO)

Medical Information*

21. Impairment Group   0008.51
                          Admission   Discharge
    Condition requiring admission to rehabilitation; code according to
    Appendix A, attached

22. Etiologic Diagnosis: OSTEOAR
    (Use ICD-9 codes to indicate the etiologic problem that led to the
    condition for which the patient is receiving rehabilitation)

23. Date of Onset of Etiologic Diagnosis   09/01/2002
                                            (MM/DD/YYYY)

24. Comorbid Conditions; Use ICD-9 Codes to enter up to ten medical
    conditions existing prior to this rehabilitation admission

    A.   B.
    C.   D.
    E.   F.
    G.   H.
    I.   J.

Medical Needs

25. Is patient comatose at admission?
                                        0 - No, 1 - Yes

26. Is patient delirious at admission?
                                        0 - No, 1 - Yes

                                        Admission Discharge

27. Swallowing Status:

    3 - *Regular Diet:* solids and liquids swallowed safely without
    supervision or modified diet

    2 - *Modified Diet/Supervision*: Subject required Modified diet and/or
    needs supervision for safety

    1 - *Tube/Parenteral Feeding:* tube / parenteral feeding used wholly or
    partially as a means of sustenance
                                        Admission Discharge

28. Clinical signs of dehydration

    (Evidence of oliguria, dru skin, orthostatic hypotension, somnolence,
    agitation; Score 0 -No; 1 - Yes)

FIGURE 13-4

Standardized assessment tools, such as the Inpatient Rehabilitation Facility–Patient assessment Instrument (IRF–PAI) shown here, can be incorporated into computerized documentation to maximize efficiency and reduce redundancy in note writing. *continued*

Function Modifiers*

Complete the following specific functional items prior to scoring the FIM Instrument:

	ADMISSION	DISCHARGE
29. Bladder Level of Assistance	07	07

Score using FIM Levels 1 - 7; 8 in unable to assess)

	ADMISSION	DISCHARGE
30. Bladder Freq. of Accidents	07	07

(Score using below)

7 - Continent
6 - Continent; uses device such as catheter
5 - Incontinent every 8 days or more
4 - Incontinent every 4 - 7 days
3 - Incontinent every 2 - 3 days; not daily
2 - Incontinent daily; some control
1 - Incontinent with every void
8 - Does not void (e.g., due to dialysis

Score Item 39G (Bladder) as the lowest (most dependent) score from Items 29 and 30 above.

	ADMISSION	DISCHARGE
31. Bowel Level of Assistance	06	06

(Score using FIM Levels 1 - 7; 8 if unable to assess)

	ADMISSION	DISCHARGE
32. Bowel Freq. of Accidents	06	06

(Score as below)

7 - Continent
6 - Continent; uses device such as ostomy
5 - Incontinent every 8 days or more
4 - Incontinent every 4 - 7 days
3 - Incontinent every 2 - 3 days; not daily
1 - Incontinent daily
8 - Could not assess, no bowel movement in 8 days

Score Item 39H (Bowel) as the lowest (most dependent) score of Items 31 and 32

	ADMISSION	DISCHARGE
33. Tub transfer	04	06
34. Shower Transfer	0	

(Score using FIM Levels 1 - 7 ; 8 if unable to assess)
Score Item 39K (Tub/Shower Transfer) as the lowest (most dependent) score of Items 33 and 34

	ADMISSION	DISCHARGE
35. Distance Walked (feet)	02	03
36. Distance Traveled Wheelchair (feet)	03	03

Score Items 35 and 36 using the following scale: 3 - 150 feet; 2 - 50 to 149 feet; 1 - Less than 50 feet or unable; 8 - Not applicable)

	ADMISSION	DISCHARGE
37. Walk	02	06
38. Wheelchair	03	03

(Score using FIM Levels 1 - 7; 8 if not applicable)
Score Item 39L (Walk,Wheelchair) as the lowest (most dependent)score of Items 37 and 38

39. FIM ™ Instrument*

SELF CARE	ADMISSION	DISCHARGE	GOAL
A. Eating	07	07	☐
B. Grooming	06	06	☐
C. Bathing	03	06	☐
D. Dressing - Upper	04	07	☐
E. Dressing - Lower	04	07	☐
F. Toileting	04	06	☐

SPHINCTER CONTROL			
G. Bladder	07	07	☐
H. Bowel	06	06	☐

TRANSFERS			
I. Bed, Chair, Whlchair	05	06	☐
J. Toilet	05	06	☐
K. Tub, Shower	04	00	☐

W - Walk
C - Wheelchair
B- - Both

LOCOMOTION			
L. Walk/Wheelchair	02 W	06 W	☐
M. Stairs	02	05	☐

A - Auditory
V - Visual
B - Both

COMMUNICATION			
N. Comprehension	04 A	07 A	☐
O. Expression	07 V	07 V	☐

V - Vocal
N - Nonvocal
B - Both

SPINAL COGNITION			
P. Social Interaction	07	07	☐
Q. Problem Solving	05	05	☐
R. Memory	07	07	☐

FIM LEVELS

No Helper

7 Complete Independence (Timely, Safely)
6 Modified Independence (Device)

Helper - Complete Dependence

5 Supervision (Subject = 100%)
4 Minimal Assistance (Subject = 75% or more)
3 Moderate Assistance (Subject = 50% or more)

Helper - Complete Dependence

2 Maximal Assistance (Subject = 25% or more)
1 Total Assistance (Subject less than 25%)

8 Activity does not occur; Use this code only at admission

FIGURE 13-4—cont'd

SUMMARY

The benefits of an automated documentation system used in a physical therapy setting (either freestanding or as part of an integrate delivery system) are numerous. Automation allows for legible, consistent standardized documentation that can be completed at the "point of care" or while the patient is present. The computer information system is a tool that can help improve consis- tency of documentation, speed and flow of information, and communication between health care providers. In addition, automation can help to decrease use of abbre- viations, integrate standardized assessment tools notes, facilitate the transfer of information to regulatory docu- ments, and facilitate data retrieval for outcomes man- agement and clinically defined "best practice" (clinical decision making) in an environment that reduces redun- dancy and error. All of these factors ultimately help to allow clinicians to spend more time with their patients.

References

Abeln S: Reporting risk check-up, *PT Magazine* 5(10): 38-42, 1997.

Adams MA, Mannion AF, Dolan P: Personal risk factors for first-time low back pain, *Spine* 23: 2497-2505, 1999.

APTA House of Delegates: *Designation "PT," "PTA," "SPT," and "SPTA,"* HOD 06-99-23-29 [Program 32] 1999.

APTA House of Delegates: *Designation by physical therapists,* HOD 06-97-06-19 [Program 32] 1997; Initial HOD 06-84-1-78 [Program

Bayley N: *Bayley Scales of Infant Development (BSID-II),* ed 2, San Antonio, Tex, 2001, Psychological Corporation.

Berg KO, Wood-Dauphinee SL, Williams JI, et al: Measuring balance in the elderly: validation of an instrument, *Can J Public Health* 83:S7-11, 1992.

Bergner M, Bobbitt RA, Carter WB, et al: The sickness impact profile: development and final revision of a health status measure, *Med Care* 19:787-805, 1981.

Bickley LS, Hoekelman RA: *JG Bates' guide to physical examination & history taking,* ed 7, Philadelphia, 1999, Lippincott Williams & Wilkins.

Bohannon RW, Smith MB: Interrater reliability of a modified Ashworth scale of muscle spasticity, *Phys Ther* 67:206-207, 1987.

Borg G, Linderholm H: Exercise performance and perceived exertion in patients with coronary insufficiency, arterial hypertension and vasoregulatory asthenia, *Acta Med Scand* 187:17-26, 1970.

Carr JH, Shepherd RB, Nordholm L, et al: Investigation of a new motor assessment scale for stroke patients, *Phys Ther* 65(2) 175-180, 1985.

Carr JH, Shepherd R: *Neurologic rehabilitation: optimizing motor performance,* Sidney, Australia, 1998, Butterworth Heinemann.

Cole AB: *Physical rehabilitation outcomes measures,* Toronto, 1995, Canadian Physiotherapy Association.

Collin C, Wade DT, Davies S, et al: The Barthel ADL Index: a reliability study, *Intern Disabil Studies* 10(2):61-63, 1988.

Coster WJ, Deeney T, Haltiwanger J, et al: *School function assessment,* San Antonio, Tex, 1998, The Psychological Corporation.

Curtis KA, Black K: Shoulder pain in female wheelchair basketball players, *J Orthop Sports Phys Ther* 29(4):225-231, 1999.

Davies GJ, Wilk A, Ellenbecker TS: Assessment of strength. In Malone TR, McPoil TG, AJ Nitz (Eds): *Orthopedic and sports physical therapy,* ed 3, St Louis, 1996, Mosby.

Davis P: *The American Heritage Dictionary of the English Language,* ed 4, New York, 2000, Houghton Mifflin.

Davis NM: *Medical abbreviations: 15,000 conveniences at the expense of communications and safety,* Huntington Valley, Penn, 2001, Neil M. Davis Associates.

*Delitto A and Snyder-Mackler L: The diagnostic process: examples in orthopedic physical therapy, *Phys Ther* 75:203-211, 1995.

Duncan PW, Weiner DK, Chandler J, et al: Functional reach: a new clinical measure of balance, *Phys Ther* 45:101-111, 1990.

Duruoz MT, Poiraudeau S, Fermanian J, et al: Development and validation of a rheumatoid hand functional disability scale that assesses functional handicap, *J Rheumatol* 23:1167-1172, 1996.

Escolar DM, Henricson EK, Mayhew J, et al: Clinical evaluator reliability for quantitative and manual muscle testing measures of strength in children, *Muscle Nerv* 24(6): 787-793, 2001.

Fairbank JCT, Couper J, Davies JB, et al: The Owestry Low Back Pain Disability Questionnaire, *Physiotherapy* 66:271-273, 1980.

Frese E, Brown M, Norton BJ: Clinical reliability of manual muscle testing: middle trapezius and gluteus medius muscles, *Physiotherapy* 67(7): 1072-1076, 1987.

Feuerstein M, Berkowitz SM, Huang GD: Predictors of occupational low back disability: implications for secondary prevention, *J Occup Environ Med* 41(12):1024-1031, 1999.

Finch E, Kennedy D: The lower extremity activity profile, *Physiotherapy Canada* 47(4):239-246, 1995.

Folio MR, Fewell RR: *Peabody developmental motor scales (PDMS-2),* ed 2, New York, 2000, Riverside Publishing.

Folstein MF, Robins LN, Helzer JE: The mini-mental state examination, *J Psychiatr Res* 12:189-198, 1975.

Fugl-Meyer A, Jaasko L, Leyman I, et al: The post-stroke hemiplegic patient: a method for evlauation of physical performance, *Scand J Rehabil Med* 6:13-31, 1975.

Gans BM, Haley SM, Hallenborg SC, et al: Description and inter-observer reliability of the Tufts assessment of motor performance, *Am J Phys Med Rehabil* 67:202-210, 1988.

Gentile AM: Skill acquisition: action, movement, and neuromotor processes. In Shepherd R, Carr J (eds): *Movement science: foundations for physical therapy in rehabilitation* Baltimore, 1987, Aspen Publishers.

Goldstein LB, Bertels C, Davis JN: Interrater reliability of the NIH stroke scale, *Arch Neurol* 46:660-662, 1989.

Guccione A: Physical therapy diagnosis and the relationship between impairment and function, *Phys Ther* (71):499-504, 1991.

Guide for the Uniform Data Set for Medical Rehabilitation (including the FIM instrument) [Computer program, version 5.0] Buffalo, 1996.

*Guide to physical therapist practice, *Phys Ther* 81(2):9-744, 2001.

Note: Items denoted with an asterisk (*) are important resources for further information pertinent to functional outcomes and documentation.

Guidelines for Physical Therapy Documentation, *Guide to physical therapist practice,* ed 2, Alexandria, Va, 2001, American Physical Therapy Association.

Guidelines for reporting and writing about people with disabilities [Brochure] Lawrence: RTC/IL, University of Kansas, 2001.

Guyatt GH, Sullivan MJ, Thompson PJ, et al: The 6-minute walk: a new measure of exercise capacity in patients with chronic heart failure, *Can Med Assoc J* (132):919-923, 1985.

Haley S, Faas R, Coster W, et al: *Pediatric evaluation of disability inventory,* Boston, 1992, New England Medical Center.

Incalzi AR, Capparella O, Gemma A, et al: A simple method of recognizing geriatric patients at risk for death and disability, *J Am Geriatr Soc* 40(1):34-38, 1992.

Jebsen RH, Taylor N, Trieschmann RB, et al: An objective and standardized test of hand function, *Arch Phys Med Rehabil* 50:311-319, 1969.

Jennett B, Teasdale G: Aspects of coma after severe head injury, *Lancet* 23(1): 878-881, 1977.

*Jette AM: Physical disablement concepts for physical therapy research and practice, *Phys Ther* 74(5):380-386, 1994.

Keith RA, Granger CV, Hamilton BB, et al: The functional independence measure: a new tool for rehabilitation: *Adv Clin Rehabil* 1:6-18, 1987.

*Kettenbach G: *Writing SOAP notes,* Philadelphia, 1995, FA Davis.

Lamb SE, Guralnik JM, Buchner DM, et al: Factors that modify the association between knee pain and mobility limitation in older women: The Women's Health and Aging Study, *Ann Rheum Dis* 59(5):331-337, 2000.

Lewis C, McNerney T: *Functional Toolbox I,* McClean, Va, 1994, Learn Publications.

Lewis C, McNerney T: *Functional Toolbox II,* McLean, Va, 1997, Learn Publications.

*Lewis K: Do the write thing: document everything! *PT Magazine* 10(7): 30-33, 2002.

Mahoney F, Barthel D: Functional evaluation: The Barthel index, *Maryland State Med J* 14:61-65, 1965.

Malone TR, McPoil TG, Nitz AJ: *Orthopedic and sports physical therapy,* ed 3, 1996, Mosby.

Martin S: Language shapes thought, *PT Magazine* May, 44-46, 1999.

Mayerson NH, Milano RA: Goniometric measurement reliability in physical medicine, *Arch Phys Med Rehabil* 65(2): 92-94, 1984.

*McEwen I: *Providing physical therapy services under parts B & C of the individuals with disabilities education act (IDEA),* Alexandria, Va, 2000, American Physical Therapy Association.

Nagi S: Some conceptual issues in disability and rehabilitation. In Sussman M (Ed): *Sociology and rehabilitation,* Washington, DC, 1965, American Sociological Association.

Nagi S: Disability concepts revisited: implication for prevention. In Pope A, Tarlov A (Eds): *Disability in America: toward a national agenda for prevention,* Washington, DC, 1991, National Academy Press.

National Advisory Board on Medical Rehabilitation Research: *Report and plan for medical rehabilitation research,* Bethesda, Md, 1991, National Institutes of Health.

O'Sullivan S, Schmitz T: *Physical rehabilitation: assessment and treatment,* Philadelphia, 2001, FA Davis.

Podsiadlo D, Richardson S: The timed "Up & Go": A test of basic functional mobility for frail elderly persons, *J Am Geriatr Soc* 39:142-148, 1991.

Randall FP, McCreary EK, Provance PG: *Muscles testing and function,* ed 4, Baltimore, 1993, Williams & Wilkins.

Randall KE, McEwen IR: Writing patient-centered functional goals, *Phys Ther* 80:1197-1203, 2000.

Reese NB, Bandy WD: *Joint range of motion and muscle length testing,* Philadelphia, 2002, WB Saunders.

Roland M, Jenner J: A revised Oswestry Disability Questionnaire. In Hudson-Cook N, Tomes-Nicholson K, Breen A (eds): *Back pain: new approaches to rehabilitation and education,* Manchester, 1989, Manchester University Press.

Scheets PK, Sahrmann SA, Norton BJ: Diagnosis for physical therapy for patients with neuromuscular conditions, *Neurology-Report* 23(4): 158-69, 1999.

*Scott RW: *Legal aspects of documenting patient care,* ed 2, Gaithersburg, Md, 2000, Aspen Publishers.

Skalko T: *Medical abbreviations for the health professions,* Ravensdale, Wash, 1998, Idyll Harbor.

*Stamer MH: *Functional documentation: a process for the physical therapist,* Tucson, 1995, Therapy Skill Builders.

Stewart AL, Hays RD, Ware JE Jr: The MOS shot general health survey: reliability and validity in a patient population, *Med Care* 26:724-735, 1988.

Stewart DL, Abeln SH: *Documenting functional outcomes in physical therapy,* St Louis, 1993, Mosby.

Stuck AE, Walthert JM, Nikolaus T, et al: Risk factors for functional status decline in community-living elderly people: a systematic literature review, *Soc Sci Med* 48:445-469, 1999.

Towle P, O'Hara D: Workbook on infant and toddler screening, evaluation and assessment, Valhalla, NY, 1995, Westchester Institute for Human Development.

Van Dillen LR, Roach KE: Reliability and validity of the Acute Care Index of Function for patients with neurologic impairment, *Phys Ther* 68(7): 1098-1101, 1988.

van Straten A, de Haan RJ, Limburg M, et al: A stroke-adapted 30-item version of the Sickness Impact Profile to assess quality of life (SA-SIP30), *Stroke* 28:2155-2161, 1997.

Vance TN: *Medicare guidelines explained for the physical therapist: a practical resource guide for physical therapy service delivery,* Gaylord, Mich, 2002, National Rehabilitation Services.

*Verbrugge L, Jette A: The disablement process, *Soc Sci Med* 38:1-14, 1994.

Westhoff G, Listing J, Zink A: Loss of physical independence in rheumatoid arthritis: interview data from a representative sample of patients in rheumatologic care, *Arthritis Care and Research* 13:11-22, 2000.

Wolf SL, Catlin PA, Gage K, et al: Establishing the reliability and validity of measurements of walking time using the Emory Functional Ambulation Profile, *Phys Ther* 79:1122-1133, 1999.

World Health Organization: *ICIDH,* 1980.

World Health Organization: *International classification of diseases (ICD-9),* New York, 1997, World Health Organization.

Guidelines for Physical Therapy Documentation

PREAMBLE

The American Physical Therapy Association (APTA) is committed to meeting the physical therapy needs of society, to meeting the needs and interest of its members, and to developing and improving the art and science of physical therapy, including practice, education, and research. To help meet these responsibilities, the APTA Board of Directors has approved the following guidelines for physical therapy documentation. It is recognized that these guidelines do not reflect all of the unique documentation requirements associated with the many specialty areas within the physical therapy profession. Applicable for both handwritten and electronic documentation systems, these guidelines are intended to be used as a foundation for the development of more specific documentation guidelines in specialty areas, while at the same time providing guidance for the physical therapy profession across all practice settings.

It is the position of APTA that physical therapy examination, evaluation, diagnosis, and prognosis shall be documented, dated, and authenticated by the physical therapist who performs the service. Intervention provided by the physical therapist or physical therapist assistant is documented, dated, and authenticated by the physical therapies or, when permissible by law, the physical therapist assistant, or both.

Other notations or flow charts are considered a component of the documented record but do not meet the requirements of documentation in, or of, themselves (Position on Authority for Physical Therapy Documentation, HOD 06-98-11-11).

OPERATIONAL DEFINITIONS

Guidelines

APTA defines "guidelines" as approved, non-binding statements of advice.

Documentation

Any entry into the client record, such as consultation report, initial examination report, progress flow, sheet/checklist that identifies the care/service provided, reexamination, or summation of care.

Authentication

The process used to verify that an entry is complete, accurate, and final. Indications of authentication can include original written signatures and computer "signatures" on secured electronic record systems only.

Adopted by the Board of Directors, APTA, March, 1993.

Amended March 2000, November 1998, March 1997, March 1995, November 1994, June 1993, March 1993.

APTA documents are revised on a regular basis. For the most recent revisions, contact www.apta.org or APTAs Service Center at 1-800-399-2782, ext. 3395.

I. GENERAL GUIDELINES

A. All documentation must comply with the applicable jurisdictional/regulatory requirements.

1. All handwritten entries shall be made in ink and will include original signatures. Electronic entries are made with appropriate security and confidentiality provisions.

2. Informed consent: The patient/client should be asked to acknowledge understanding and consent before intervention is initiated.

    Examples of ways in which to accomplish this documentation:

    Ex. 2.1   Signature of patient/client or parent/legal guardian on long or short consent form.

    Ex. 2.2   Notation/entry of what was explained by the physical therapist in the official record.

    Ex. 2.3   Filing of a completed consent checklist signed by the patient/client or parent/legal guardian.

3. Charting errors should be corrected by drawing a single lines through the error and initialing and dating the chart or through the appropriate mechanism for electronic documentation that clearly indicates that a change was made without deletion of the original record.

4. Identification.

    4.1   Include patient/client's full name and identification number, if applicable, on all official documents.

    4.2   All entries must be dated and authenticated with the provider's full name and appropriate designation (i.e., PT or PTA)

    4.3   Documentation by graduates or others pending receipt of an unrestricted license shall be authenticated by a licensed physical therapist.

    4.4   Documentation by students (SPT/SPTA) in physical therapist or physical therapist assistant programs must be additionally authenticated by the physical therapist or, when permissible by law, documentation by physical therapist assistant students may be authenticated by a physical therapist assistant.

5. Documentation should include the referral mechanism by which physical therapy services are initiated.
   Examples include:

    Ex. 5.1   Self-referral/direct access.

    Ex. 5.2   Request for consultation from a practitioner.

II. INITIAL EXAMINATION AND EVALUATION/CONSULTATION

A. Documentation is required at the outset of each episode of physical therapy care.

B. Documentation of the initial episode of physical therapy shall include the following elements:

1. Documentation of appropriate history:

    1.1   History of the presenting problem, current complaints, and precautions (including onset date).

    1.2   Pertinent diagnoses and medical history.

    1.3   Demographic characteristics, including pertinent psychological, social, and environmental factors.

    1.4   Prior or concurrent services related to the current episode of physical therapy care.

    1.5   Comorbidities that may affect prognosis.

    1.6   Statement of patient/client's knowledge or problem.

    1.7   Anticipated goals of and expected outcomes for the patient/client (and family members, or significant others, if appropriate).

2. Documentation of a systems review

    2.1   Documentation of physiologic and anatomical status to include the following systems:

    2.1.1   Cardiovascular/pulmonary
    2.1.2   Integumentary
    2.1.3   Musculoskeletal
    2.1.4   Neuromuscular

    2.2   A review of communication, affect, cognition, language, and learning style.

3. Documentation of selection and administration of appropriate tests and measures to determine patient/client status in a number of areas and documentation of findings. The following is a partial list of these areas to be addressed in the documented examination and evaluation, including illustrative tests and measures:

    3.1   Arousal, mentation, and cognition

    Examples include objective findings related, but not limited, to the following areas:

    Ex. 3.1.1   Level of consciousness
    Ex. 3.1.2   Ability to process commands
    Ex. 3.1.3   Gross expressive deficits

    3.2   Neuromotor development and sensory integration

    Examples include examination findings related, but not limited, to the following areas:

Ex. 3.2.1 Gross and fine motor skills
Ex. 3.2.2 Reflex and movement patterns
Ex. 3.2.3 Dexterity, agility, and coordination

3.3 Range of motion

Examples include objective findings related, but not limited, to the following areas:

Ex. 3.3.1 Extent of joint motion
Ex. 3.3.2 Pain and soreness of surrounding soft tissue
Ex. 3.3.3 Muscle length and flexibility

3.4 Muscle performance (including strength, power, and endurance)

Examples include objective findings related, but not limited, to the following areas:

Ex. 3.4.1 Force, velocity, torque, work, power
Ex. 3.4.2 Manual muscle test grades
Ex. 3.4.3 Amplitude, duration, waveform, and frequency of electromyographic (EMG) signals

3.5 Ventilation, respiration (gas exchange), and circulation

Examples include objective findings related, but not limited, to the following areas:

Ex. 3.5.1 Heart rate (HR), respiratory rate (RR), blood pressure (BP)
Ex. 3.5.2 Arterial blood gases
Ex. 3.5.3 Palpation of peripheral pulses

3.6 Posture

Examples include objective findings related, but not limited, to the following areas:

Ex. 3.6.1 Static posture
Ex. 3.6.2 Dynamic posture

3.7 Gait, locomotion, and balance

Examples include objective findings related, but not limited, to the following areas:

Ex. 3.7.1 Characteristics of gait
Ex. 3.7.2 Functional ambulation
Ex. 3.7.3 Characteristics of balance

3.8 Self-care and home management

Examples include objective findings related, but not limited, to the following areas:

Ex. 3.8.1 Activities of daily living
Ex. 3.8.2 Functional capacity
Ex. 3.8.3 Transfers

3.9 Community and work (job/school/play) integration or reintegration

Ex. 3.9.1 Instrumental activities of daily living
Ex. 3.9.2 Functional capacity
Ex. 3.9.3 Adaptive skills

4. Documentation of evaluation (a dynamic process in which the physical therapist makes clinical judgments based on data gathered during the examination).

5. Documentation of diagnosis (a label encompassing a cluster of signs and symptoms, syndromes, or categories that reflects the information obtained from the examination).

6. Documentation of prognosis (determination of the level of optimal improvement that might be attained through intervention and the amount of time required to reach that level. Documentation shall include anticipated goals, expected outcomes, and plan of care).

6.1 Patient/client (and family members or significant others, if appropriate) is involved in establishing anticipated goals and expected outcomes.

6.2 All anticipated goals and expected outcomes are stated in measurable terms.

6.3 Anticipated goals and expected outcomes are related to impairments, functional limitations, and disabilities identified in the examination.

6.4 All expected outcomes are stated in functional terms.

6.5 The plan of care:

6.5.1 Is related to anticipated goals and expected outcomes.

6.5.2 Includes frequency and duration to achieve the anticipated goals and expected outcomes.

6.5.3 Includes patient/client and family/caregiver educational goals.

6.5.4 Involves appropriate collaboration and coordination of care with other professionals/services.

7. Authentication by and appropriate designation of physical therapist.

III. DOCUMENTATION OF THE CONTINUUM OF CARE

A. Documentation of intervention or services provided and current patient/client status.

1. Documentation is required for each patient visit/encounter.

1.1 Authentication and appropriate designation of the physical therapist of physical therapist assistant providing the service under the supervision of the physical therapist.

2. Documentation of each visit/encounter shall include the following elements:

   2.1 Patient/client self-reports (as appropriate).

   2.2 Identification of specific interventions provided, including frequency, intensity, and duration as appropriate.

   Examples include:

   Ex. 2.2.1 Knee extensions, 3 sets, 10 repetitions, 10-lb weight
   Ex. 2.2.2 Transfer training bed to chair with sliding board

   2.3 Equipment provided.
   2.4 Changes in patient/client status as they relate to the plan of care.
   2.5 Adverse reactions to interventions, in any.
   2.6 Factors that modify frequency of intensity of intervention and progression towards anticipated goals, including patient/client adherence to patient/client-related instructions.
   2.7 Communication/consultation with providers/patient/client/family/significant other.

B. Documentation of Reexamination
   1. Documentation of reexamination is provided as appropriate to evaluate progress and to modify or redirect intervention.
   2. Documentation of reexamination shall include the following elements:

      2.1 Documentation of elements as identified in III.A.2 to update patient/client/s status.
      2.2 Interpretation of findings and, when indicated, revision of anticipated goals and expected outcomes.
      2.3 When indicated, revision of plan of care as directly correlated wit anticipated goals and expected outcomes as documented.
      2.4 Authentication by and appropriate designation of the physical therapist.

IV. DOCUMENTATION OF SUMMATION OF EPISODE OF CARE

A. Documentation is required following conclusion of the current episode in the physical therapy intervention sequence.
B. Documentation of the summation of the episode of care shall include the following elements:
   1. Criteria for discharge

   Examples include:

   Ex. 1.1 Anticipated goals and expected outcomes have been achieved.
   Ex. 1.2 Patient/client, caregiver, or legal guardian declines to continue intervention.
   Ex. 1.3 Patient/client is unable to continue to work toward anticipated goals due to medical or psychosocial complications.
   Ex. 1.4 Physical therapist determines that the patient/client will no longer benefit from physical therapy.

   2. Current physical/functional status.
   3. Degree of anticipated goal and expected outcome achieved and reasons for goals and outcomes not being achieved.
   4. Discharge plan that includes written and verbal communication related to the patient/client's continuing care.

   Examples include:

   Ex. 4.1 Home program.
   Ex. 4.2 Referrals for additional services.
   Ex. 4.3 Recommendations for follow-up physical therapy care.
   Ex. 4.4 Family and caregiver training.
   Ex. 4.5 Equipment provided.

   5. Authentication and appropriate designation of physical therapist.

Additional References

1. *Direction and Supervision of the Physical Therapist Assistant.* (HOD 06-99-30-42).
2. *Comprehensive Accreditation Manual for Hospitals.* Oakbrook Terrace, Ill: Joint Commission on Accreditation of Healthcare Organizations; 1996.
3. *Glossary of Terms Related to Information Security.* Schaumburg, Ill: Computer-based Patient Record Institute; 1996.
4. *Guidelines for Establishing Information Security Policies at Organizations Using Computed-based Patient Records.* Schaumburg, Ill: Computer-Based Record Institute; 1995.
5. *Current Procedural Terminology.* Chicago: American Medical Association (AMA); 2000.
6. *Coding and Payment Guide for the Physical Therapist.* Washington, DC: St. Anthony's Publishing; 2000.
7. *Minimal Data Set (MDS) Regulations.* Healthcare Financing Administration (HCFA). Available at: www.hcfa.gov
8. *HCFA/AMA Documentation Guidelines.* Healthcare Financing Administration (HCFA). Available at: www.hcfa.gov
9. *Home Health Regulations.* Healthcare Financing Administration (HCFA). Available at: www.hcfa.gov
10. State Practice Acts. Available at: www.fsbpt.org

Rehabilitation Abbreviations

The following list of abbreviation is divided into the following categories: general, professional, medical diagnosis, and symbols. In addition, this entire list (categories combined) is organized alphabetically in reverse order (by word versus abbreviation).

GENERAL

A or Ⓐ	assistance
A	assessment
AAA	abdominal aortic aneurysm
AAFO	articulating ankle foot orthosis
AAROM	active assistive range of motion
Abd or ABD	abduction
ABG	arterial blood gases
abn	abnormal
AC	alternating current
ACA	anterior cerebral artery
ACL	anterior cruciate ligament
AD	assistive device
Add or ADD	adduction
ADL	activities of daily living
ad lib	at discretion
Afib	atrial fibrillation
AFO	ankle foot orthosis
AG	against gravity
AK	above knee
amb	ambulatory, ambulation
ant	anterior
AP	anteroposterior
approx	approximate, approximately
appt	appointment
A&O	alert and oriented
AROM	active range of motion
ASIA	American Spinal Injury Association
ASIS	anterior superior iliac spine

assist	assistant, assistance
ATNR	assymetrical tonic neck reflex
AV	atrioventricular
B or Ⓑ	bilateral
B&B	bowel and bladder
bal	balance
BE	below elbow
b.i.d.	twice a day
bil	bilateral
b.i.w.	biweekly
BK	below knee
BM	bowel movement
BNL	below normal limits
BOS	base of support
BP	blood pressure
bpm	beats per minute
BS	breath sounds
$\bar{c}$	with
CICU	cardiac intensive care unit
CG	contact guarding
cm	centimeter
CNS	central nervous system
c/o	complained of, complains of
cont'd	continued
CO_2	carbon dioxide
CPAP	continuous positive airway pressure
CPT	chest physical therapy
CS	close supervision
CSF	cerebrospinal fluid
CT	computed tomography
d	day
D	dependent
DAI	diffuse axonal injury
DBE	deep breathing exercise
D/C	discharge; discontinue
Dep	dependent
DF	dorsiflexion
DIP	distal interphalangeal (joint)
dist	distance, distant
DME	durable medical equipment
DS	distant supervision
DTR	deep tendon reflex
dx	diagnosis

Adapted from Burke Rehabilitation Hospital, White Plains, New York.

ECF	extended care facility	LLB	long leg brace
ECG	electrocardiogram	LLE	left lower extremity
EEG	electroencephalogram	LLL	left lower lobe
EKG	electrocardiogram	LLQ	left lower quadrant
EMG	electromyogram	lig(s)	ligament(s)
ENT	ear, nose, throat	LOB	loss of balance
equip	equipment	LOC	loss of consciousness
ER	emergency room; external rotation	L/min	liters per minute
e-stim	electrical stimulation	LTG	long-term goal(s)
eval	evaluation	LTC	long-term care
ex	exercise	LTM	long-term memory
exam	examination	LUE	left upper extremity
ext	external; extension	LUL	left upper lobe
ext rot, ER	external rotation	LUQ	left upper quadrant
F	fair (muscle grade)	LVH	left ventricular hypertrophy
FES	functional electric stimulation	m	meters
flex	flexion	max	maximal, maximum
freq	frequently, frequency	MCA	middle cerebral artery
F/U	follow-up	MCP	metacarpophalangeal joint
FWB	full weight bearing	med	medical
Fx	function, fracture	MH	moist heat
G	good (muscle grade)	min	minute(s), minimal
GCS	Glasgow Coma Scale	MMT	manual muscle test
GE	gravity eliminated	mod	moderate
GI	gastrointestinal	MRI	magnetic resonance imaging
G-tube	gastrostomy tube	MVA	motor vehicle accident
h	hour	mvt	movement
HA	headache	N	normal (muscle grade)
HEP	home exercise program	N/A	not applicable
HHA	home health aide	n/avail	not available
H/O	history of	NBQC	narrow-based quad cane
HOH	hard of hearing	Neg	negative
HR	heart rate	NG	nasogastric
HTN	hypertension	NICU	neonatal intensive care unit
hx	history	NPO	nothing by mouth
H_2O	water	N/T	not tested
I or Ind	independent	NWB	non–weight-bearing
I&O	intake and output	OOB	out of bed
ICU	intensive care unit	OR	operating room
inf	inferior	ORIF	open reduction internal fixation
int	internal	O_2	oxygen
int rot, IR	internal rotation	p̄	after
IQ	intelligence quotient	Ⓟ	poor (muscle grade)
IV	intravenous	PA	posterior anterior
jt	joint	PCA	posterior cerebral artery
J-tube	jejunostomy tube	PET	positron emission tomography
K	potassium	PF	plantar flexion
KAFO	knee ankle foot orthosis	PIP	proximal interphalangeal (joint)
KCAL	kilocalorie	PLS	posterior leaf splint
kg	kilogram(s)	PMH	past medical history
L or Ⓛ	left or liter	PO	by mouth
lat	lateral	post	posterior
lb	pound	post op	postoperative
LBP	lower back pain	PRE	progressive resistive exercise(s)
LBQC	large-based quad cane	prn	as often as necessary
LE	lower extremity	PROM	passive range of motion

prox	proximal
PRW	platform rolling walker
PSH	past surgical history
PSIS	posterior superior iliac spine
PTA	prior to admission
Pt	patient
P&V	percussion and vibration
PWB	partial weight-bearing
q	every
q.i.d.	every day
quads	quadriceps
R or Ⓡ	right
re	concerning, regarding
rehab	rehabilitation
reps	repetitions
RLE	right lower extremity
RLL	right lower lobe
RLQ	right lower quadrant
RML	right middle lobe
R/O	rule out, ruled out
ROM	range of motion
RR	respiratory rate
RROM	resisted range of motion
R/T	related to
RUE	right upper extremity
RUL	right upper lobe
RUQ	right upper quadrant
RW	rolling walker
Rx	prescription; treatment; orders
S or Ⓢ	supervision
s̄	without
SAQ	short arc quads
SB	sliding board
SBA	stand by assistance
SBQC	small-based quad cane
SBT	sliding board transfers
SCM	sternocleidomastoid muscle
sec	second(s)
sig	significant
SLR	straight leg raise
SNF	skilled nursing facility
S/O	standing order
SOB	shortness of breath
SOS	step-over-step (stair climbing)
s/p	status post
SPT	stand pivot transfers
staph	Staphylococcus
stat	immediately, at once
STG	short-term goal(s)
STM	short-term memory
STNR	symmetrical tonic neck reflex
str cane	straight cane
strep	Streptococcus
STS	sit to stand; step-to-step (stair climbing)
supp	supported
surg	surgical, surgery

sx	symptoms
symm	symmetrical, symmetry
T	trace (muscle grade)
TBA	to be assessed
TBE	to be evaluated
TDWB	touch down weight bearing
temp	temperature
TENS	transcutaneous electrical nerve stimulator
ther ex	therapeutic exercise
t.i.w.	three times per week
TMJ	temporomandibular joint
T/O	throughout
TOL	tolerate(s)
TR	transfer
trach	tracheostomy
trans	transverse, transferred
trng	training
TTWB	toe touch weight bearing
Tx	treatment
UE	upper extremity
U/L	unilateral
unsupp	unsupported
URI	upper respiratory infection
US	ultrasound
UTI	urinary tract infection
VAS	visual analog scale
VC	verbal cues, vital capacity, vocal cord
V/O	verbal order
VS	vital signs
Vtach	ventricular tachycardia
WB	weight bearing
WBAT	weight bearing as tolerated
WBQC	wide-based quad cane
W/C	wheelchair
WFL	within functional limits
WNL	within normal limits
WS	weight shift
wk	week(s)
x	times (i.e., $6 \times d$ = six times daily); for (i.e., $\times 5$ yrs = for 5 yrs); of (i.e., 3 sets x 10 reps)
x̄	except
y/o or y.o.	years old

PROFESSIONALS

ATC	Athletic Trainer Certified
CCC-A	Certificate of Clinical Competence—Audiology
CCC-SLP	Certificate of Clinical Competence—Speech, Language Pathology
CDN	Certified Dietitian
CFY-SLP	Clinical Fellowship Year—Speech, Language Pathology

CNA	Certified Nursing Assistant
COTA	Certified Occupational Therapy Assistant
CSW	Certified Social Worker
CTRS	Certified Therapeutic Recreation Specialist
CRTT	Certified Respiratory Therapy Technician
DTR	Registered Dietetic Technician
GYN	gynecological, gynecology
HHA	Home Health Aide
LPN	Licensed Practical Nurse
MD	Medical Doctor
MSW	Master of Social Work
OB	obstetrics
OT	Occupational Therapy
OTOL	otolaryngology
OTR	Occupational Therapist Registered
OTR/L	Occupational Therapist Registered/Licensed
PED	pediatrics, pediatrician
PA	Physician's Assistant
PT	Physical Therapist, Physical Therapy
PTA	Physical Therapist Assistant
RD	Registered Dietitian
RN	Registered Nurse
RRT	Registered Respiratory Therapist
SLP	Speech Language Pathologist
TR	Therapeutic Recreation

GBS	Guillain-Barré syndrome
GSW	gunshot wound
HD	Huntington's disease
HIV	human immunodeficiency virus
IDDM	insulin-dependent diabetes mellitus—Type I
MI	myocardial infarction
MS	multiple sclerosis
NIDDM	non–insulin-dependent diabetes mellitus—Type II
OA	osteoarthritis
OBS	organic brain syndrome
PD	Parkinson's disease
PSP	progressive supranuclear palsy
PVD	peripheral vascular disease
RA	rheumatoid arthritis
SAH	subarachnoid hemorrhage
SCI	spinal cord injury
TB	tuberculosis
TBI	traumatic brain injury
THI	traumatic head injury
THR	total hip replacement
TIA	transient ischemic attack
TKR	total knee replacement
TSR	total shoulder replacement

MEDICAL DIAGNOSES

ADD	attention deficit disorder without hyperactivity
ADHD	attention deficit hyperactivity disorder
AIDS	acquired immunodeficiency syndrome
AKA	above knee amputation
ALS	amyotrophic lateral sclerosis
ASD	arterial septal defect
ASHD	arteriosclerotic heart disease
AVM	arteriovenous malformation
BKA	below-knee amputation
CA	carcinoma
CABG	coronary artery bypass graft
CAD	coronary artery disease
CFS	chronic fatigue syndrome
CHF	congestive heart failure
CHI	closed head injury
COPD	chronic obstructive pulmonary disease
CVA	cerebrovascular accident
DVT	deep vein thrombosis
DJD	degenerative joint disease

SYMBOLS

1°	initial, primary, first degree
2°	secondary, second degree
3°	tertiary, third degree
=	equal
≠	not equal
−	negative, minus, inhibitory
+	positive, plus, facilitory
>	greater than
<	less than
/	extension, extensor
✓	flexion, flexor
♀	female
♂	male
‖	parallel
@	at
Δ	change
↑	increase, up, improve
↓	decrease, down, decline
←→	to and from
#	pound, number

ABBREVIATIONS BY WORD

abdominal aortic aneurysm	AAA
abduction	Abd or ABD
abnormal	abn
above knee	AK
above knee amputation	AKA
acquired immunodeficiency syndrome	AIDS
active assistive range of motion	AAROM
active range of motion	AROM
activities of daily living	ADL
adduction	Add or ADD
after	$\bar{p}$
against gravity	AG
alert and oriented	A&O
alternating current	AC
ambulatory, ambulation	amb
American Spinal Injury Association	ASIA
amyotrophic lateral sclerosis	ALS
ankle foot orthosis	AFO
anterior	ant
anterior cerebral artery	ACA
anterior cruciate ligament	ACL
anterior superior iliac spine	ASIS
anteroposterior	AP
appointment	appt
approximate, approximately	approx
arterial blood gases	ABG
atrial septal defect	ASD
arteriosclerotic heart disease	ASHD
arteriovenous malformation	AVM
articulating ankle foot orthosis	AAFO
as often as necessary	prn
assessment	A
assistance	A or Ⓐ
assistant, assistance	assist
assistive device	AD
asymmetrical tonic neck reflex	ATNR
at	@
at discretion	ad lib
Athletic Trainer Certified	ATC
atrial fibrillation	Afib
atrioventricular	AV
attention deficit disorder without hyperactivity	ADD
attention deficit hyperactivity disorder	ADHD
balance	bal
base of support	BOS
beats per minute	bpm
below elbow	BE
below knee	BK
below-knee amputation	BKA
below normal limits	BNL
bilateral	bil, B, or Ⓑ
biweekly	b.i.w.
blood pressure	BP
bowel and bladder	B&B
bowel movement	BM
breath sounds	BS
by mouth	PO
carbon dioxide	CO_2
carcinoma	CA
cardiac intensive care unit	CICU
centimeter	cm
central nervous system	CNS
cerebrovascular accident	CVA
cerebrospinal fluid	CSF
Certificate of Clinical Competence—Audiology	CCC-A
Certificate of Clinical Competence—Speech, Language Pathology	CCC-SLP
Certified Dietitian	CDN
Certified Nursing Assistant	CNA
Certified Occupational Therapy Assistant	COTA
Certified Respiratory Therapy Technician	CRTT
Certified Social Worker	CSW
Certified Therapeutic Recreation Specialist	CTRS
change	Δ
chest physical therapy	CPT
chronic fatigue syndrome	CFS
chronic obstructive pulmonary disease	COPD
Clinical Fellowship Year—Speech, Language Pathology	CFY-SLP
close supervision	CS
closed head injury	CHI
complained of, complains of	c/o
computed tomography	CT
congestive heart failure	CHF
contact guarding	CG
continued	cont'd
continuous positive airway pressure	CPAP
coronary artery bypass graft	CABG
coronary artery disease	CAD
day	d
decrease, down, decline	↓
deep breathing exercise	DBE
deep tendon reflex	DTR
deep vein thrombosis	DVT
degenerative joint disease	DJD
dependent	D, dep
diagnosis	dx
diffuse axonal injury	DAI
discharge	D/C
discontinue	D/C
distal interphalangeal (joint)	DIP
distance, distant	dist
distant supervision	DS
dorsiflexion	DF
durable medical equipment	DME

ear, nose, throat	ENT	inhibitory	−
electrical stimulation	e-stim	initial	1°
electrocardiogram	ECG, EKG	insulin-dependent diabetes	
electroencephalogram	EEG	mellitus—Type I	IDDM
electromyogram	EMG	intake and output	I&O
emergency room	ER	intelligence quotient	IQ
equal	=	intensive care unit	ICU
equipment	equip	internal	int
evaluation	eval	internal rotation	int rot, IR
every	q	intravenous	IV
every day	q.i.d.	improve	↑
examination	exam	jejunostomy tube	J-tube
except	x̄	joint	jt
exercise	ex	kilocalorie	KCAL
extended care facility	ECF	kilogram(s)	kg
extension	ext, /	knee ankle foot orthosis	KAFO
extensor	/	large-based quad cane	LBQC
external	ext	lateral	lat
external rotation	ext rot, ER	left or liter	L or Ⓛ
facilitory	+	left lower extremity	LLE
fair (muscle grade)	F	left lower lobe	LLL
female	♀	left lower quadrant	LLQ
first degree	1°	left upper extremity	LUE
flexion	flex, ✓	left upper lobe	LUL
flexor	✓	left upper quadrant	LUQ
follow-up	F/U	left ventricular hypertrophy	LVH
for (i.e., × 5 yrs = for 5 yrs)	×	less than	<
fracture	Fx	Licensed Practical Nurse	LPN
frequently, frequency	freq	ligament(s)	lig(s)
full weight bearing	FWB	liters	L
function	Fx	liters per minute	L/min
functional electric stimulation	FES	long leg brace	LLB
gastrointestinal	GI	long-term goal(s)	LTG
gastrostomy tube	G-tube	long-term care	LTC
Glasgow Coma Scale	GCS	long-term memory	LTM
good (muscle grade)	G	loss of balance	LOB
gravity eliminated	GE	loss of consciousness	LOC
greater than	>	lower back pain	LBP
Guillain-Barré syndrome	GBS	lower extremity	LE
gunshot wound	GSW	magnetic resonance imaging	MRI
gynecology	GYN	male	♂
hard of hearing	HOH	manual muscle test	MMT
headache	HA	Master of Social Work	MSW
heart rate	HR	maximal, maximum	max
history	hx	medical	med
history of	H/O	Medical Doctor	MD
home exercise program	HEP	metacarpophalangeal joint	MCP
home health aide	HHA	meters	m
hour	h	middle cerebral artery	MCA
human immunodeficiency virus	HIV	minus	−
Huntington's disease	HD	minute(s), minimal	min
hypertension	HTN	moderate	mod
immediately, at once	stat	moist heat	MH
increase, up, improve	↑	motor vehicle accident	MVA
independent	I or Ind	movement	mvt
inferior	inf	multiple sclerosis	MS

myocardial infarction	MI	primary	1°
narrow-based quad cane	NBQC	prior to admission	PTA
nasogastric	NG	progressive resistive exercise(s)	PRE
negative	–, Neg	progressive supranuclear palsy	PSP
neonatal intensive care unit	NICU	proximal	prox
non–insulin-dependent diabetes		proximal interphalangeal (joint)	PIP
mellitus—Type II	NIDDM	quadriceps	quads
non–weight-bearing	NWB	range of motion	ROM
normal (muscle grade)	N	regarding, concerning	re
not applicable	N/A	Registered Dietitian	RD
not available	n/avail	Registered Nurse	RN
not equal	≠	Registered Respiratory Therapist	RRT
not tested	N/T	Registered Dietetic Technician	DTR
nothing by mouth	NPO	rehabilitation	rehab
number	#	related to	R/T
obstetrics	OB	repetitions	reps
Occupational Therapy	OT	resisted range of motion	RROM
Occupational Therapist Registered	OTR	respiratory rate	RR
Occupational Therapist		rheumatoid arthritis	RA
Registered/Licensed	OTR/L	right	R or Ⓡ
of (i.e., 3 sets × 10 reps)	×	right lower extremity	RLE
open reduction internal fixation	ORIF	right lower lobe	RLL
operating room	OR	right lower quadrant	RLQ
orders	Rx	right middle lobe	RML
organic brain syndrome	OBS	right upper extremity	RUE
osteoarthritis	OA	right upper lobe	RUL
otolaryngology	OTOL	right upper quadrant	RUQ
out of bed	OOB	rolling walker	RW
oxygen	O$_2$	rule out, ruled out	R/O
parallel	||	second(s)	sec
Parkinson's disease	PD	secondary, second degree	2°
partial weight-bearing	PWB	short arc quads	SAQ
passive range of motion	PROM	shortness of breath	SOB
past medical history	PMH	short-term goal(s)	STG
past surgical history	PSH	short-term memory	STM
patient	Pt	significant	sig
pediatrics	PED	sit to stand	STS
percussion and vibration	P&V	skilled nursing facility	SNF
peripheral vascular disease	PVD	sliding board	SB
Physician's Assistant	PA	sliding board transfers	SBT
Physical Therapist, Physical Therapy	PT	small-based quad cane	SBQC
Physical Therapist Assistant	PTA	Speech Language Pathologist	SLP
plantar flexion	PF	spinal cord injury	SCI
platform rolling walker	PRW	stand by assistance	SBA
poor (muscle grade)	Ⓟ	stand pivot transfers	SPT
positive, plus	+	standing order	S/O
posterior	post	Staphylococcus	staph
posterior anterior	PA	status post	s/p
posterior cerebral artery	PCA	step-over-step (stair climbing)	SOS
positron emission tomography	PET	step-to-step (stair climbing)	STS
posterior leaf splint	PLS	sternocleidomastoid muscle	SCM
posterior superior iliac spine	PSIS	straight cane	str cane
postoperative	post op	straight leg raise	SLR
potassium	K	Streptococcus	strep
pound	lb, #	subarachnoid hemorrhage	SAH
prescription	Rx	supervision	S or Ⓢ

supported	supp	traumatic head injury	THI
surgical, surgery	surg	treatment	Tx, Rx
symmetric, symmetry	symm	tuberculosis	TB
symmetrical tonic neck relfex	STNR	twice a day	b.i.d.
symptoms	sx	ultrasound	US
temperature	temp	unilateral	U/L
temporomandibular joint	TMJ	unsupported	unsupp
tertiary	3°	upper extremity	UE
therapeutic exercise	ther ex	upper respiratory infection	URI
Therapeutic Recreation	TR	urinary tract infection	UTI
third degree	3°	ventricular tachycardia	Vtach
three times per week	t.i.w.	verbal cues	VC
throughout	T/O	verbal order	V/O
times (i.e., 6×d = six times daily	×	visual analog scale	VAS
to and from	←→	vital capacity	VC
to be assessed	TBA	vital signs	VS
to be evaluated	TBE	vocal cord	VC
toe touch weight bearing	TTWB	water	H_2O
total hip replacement	THR	week(s)	wk
total knee replacement	TKR	weight bearing	WB
total shoulder replacement	TSR	weight bearing as tolerated	WBAT
touch down weight bearing	TDWB	weight shift	WS
trace (muscle grade)	T	wheelchair	W/C
tracheostomy	trach	wide-based quad cane	WBQC
training	trng	with	c̄
transcutaneous electrical nerve stimulator	TENS	within functional limits	WFL
transfer	TR	within normal limits	WNL
transient ischemic attack	TIA	without	s̄
transverse, transferred	trans	years old	y/o or y.o.
traumatic brain injury	TBI		

Answers to Exercises

1. **I**—Range of motion is at impairment level. Musculoskeletal flexibility is measured in units of joint rotation.

2. **F**—Patient's ability to walk is generally measured at the functional level. Performance of whole person is measured.

3. **P**—Medical diagnosis specifying location and type of tissue damage.

4. **D**—Patient's ability to fulfill occupational role is at disability level.

5. **I**—Strength is a measure of impairment.

6. **F**—Dressing is a functional activity.

7. **P**—This is a medical diagnosis that specifies the location and nature of tissue damage.

8. **I**—Even though the functional activity of stair climbing is referred to, the observation is of the patient's cardiopulmonary function, a description of the function of a body system. The emphasis of this statement is on the cardiopulmonary function.

9. **P**—Multiple sclerosis describes a type of brain disease. The cause is not yet known. This is a medical diagnosis.

10. **F**—Eating is a functional activity. Here the word *independently* is used, specifying how the performance is achieved. Even though this term may also be used in reference to disability, here the emphasis is on performance of a specific functional activity.

11. **I**—Lateral pinch strength is an impairment. Here it describes a body function of a body system (musculoskeletal).

12. **F**—Transfers are functional activities described here in terms of goal attainment and with use of adaptive equipment (sliding board).

13. **I**—Passive range of motion is an impairment.

14. **F**—Reaching and grasping a cup is a functional task.

15. **F**—Standing at a kitchen sink is an important functional activity.

16. **I**—A straight leg raise reflects performance of a body system (musculoskeletal). This is a way of specifying active range of motion.

17. **I**—Pain is considered an impairment. A functional activity is not mentioned.

18. **D**—Daily household chores describe a range of activities that encompass a person's disability related to his or her personal roles in life. Overall level of assistance, or caregiver burden, reflects a disability.

19. **F**—Cooking and preparing dinner are specific functional skills.

20. **F**—Getting in and out of a wheelchair is an important functional skill for a person who uses a wheelchair for mobility.

21. **P**—A spinal cord injury is a specific pathologic condition; the MVA specifies the mechanism of injury.

22. **D**—Accessibility to a person's community encompasses that person's disability. It is a global measure, rather than specifically identifying his or her functional skill in wheelchair mobility, for example.

23. **P**—A rotator cuff tear is a pathologic condition of the shoulder.

24. **D**—Returning to work represents a component of a person's disability (occupational role).

25. **F**—Walking is an important functional skill.

CHAPTER 2

EXERCISE 2-1*

1. *A quadriplegic will require help with transfers.*
   Quadriplegic is a label that reduces an individual to a disability or physical condition. Try patient with quadriplegia (or, if the person in question is not currently receiving care, person with quadriplegia). Terms such as *quad* should never be used to refer to a person.

2. *The patient was afflicted with multiple sclerosis when she was in her 20s.*
   Expressions such as *afflicted with, suffers from,* or *is a victim of* sensationalize a person's health status and may be considered patronizing. Simply say the patient was first diagnosed with multiple sclerosis in her 20s or that the patient developed the condition.

3. *Many PTs are involved in foot clinics for diabetics.*
   Here again, the problem is a label. Consider " ... foot clinics for people with diabetes."

4. *Have you finished the documentation for that shoulder in room 316?*
   Unbelievable as it may seem, some health care providers still can be heard referring to patients as body parts. This question could easily be reworded as "Have you finished the documentation for the patient in room 316 with shoulder pain?"

5. *The patient complained of pain in the right upper extremity.*
   Complaining of may suggest that the patient is overreacting to his or her symptoms or is difficult to work with. Instead, say the patient reported the pain.

6. *A care plan for a total knee patient typically involves a strong element of patient education.*
   Suggested: "A care plan for a patient with a total knee replacement...." Putting the patient first emphasizes the person, not his or her health status.

7. *Although this computer program was designed for the disabled, able-bodied users will also find it helpful.*
   Not only is *disabled* a label when used to describe a person with disabilities, in this sentence it also has the effect of grouping the individual into a distinct "disability class." In addition, use of the term *able-bodied* (as well as *healthy* or *whole*) to contrast people without disabilities with people who have disabilities is considered inappropriate. Better: "Although this computer program was designed for people with disabilities, users without disabilities will also find it helpful."

8. *Because of a spinal cord injury, the patient was confined to a wheelchair.*
   To a person who lives an active, full life with the use of a wheelchair, *confined to* can have a patronizing ring; consider saying "...the patient uses a wheelchair."

9. *Nine of 10 patients receiving physical therapy expressed interest in a group exercise session.*
   Appropriate.

10. *The patient is behaving like a child.*
    This has a negative connotation and is derogatory. Statements should be kept to objective facts (e.g., stating what the patient's behavior was, rather than interpreting it).

11. *Which therapist is treating the brain-injured patient in room 216?*
    People-first language should be used. "Patient with a brain injury."

*Some answers are adapted with permission from Martin (Martin, 1999).

12. *The stroke victim can often return to work.*
    Patients are not *victims*. Restate as "A person who has had a stroke can often return to work."

13. *The patient refused to modify her footwear choice even after the therapist told her not to wear 2-inch heels.*
    Refused may be too strong a word. Restate as "Following a discussion of heel height, the patient reported she felt no need to modify her heel height choice."

14. *I'll put my 10:00 on the machine while my 10:15 gets a hot pack.*
    Patients have names and it is important to use them or at least refer to patients as people.

15. *The patient suffers from Parkinson's disease.*
    This implies that people with Parkinson's disease (or other diseases) suffer in some way, which is not always the case. Restate as "Mr. Jones has a diagnosis of Parkinson's disease."

EXERCISE 2-2

1. Manual muscle test 3/5 right quadriceps.

2. Patient can stand without assistance for 30 seconds without loss of balance.

3. Patient can transfer from bed to wheelchair with moderate assistance using sliding board.

4. Patient instructed in performing right short arc quads, 3 sets of 10 repetitions.

5. Passive range of motion of right ankle dorsiflexion 5 degrees.

6. Received order from (patient's) medical doctor for weight bearing as tolerated on left lower extremity.

7. Patient instructed to perform home exercise program twice a day, 10 repetitions each exercise.

8. Patient admitted to emergency room on 10/12/00 with Glasgow Coma Scale score of 4.

9. Medical diagnosis: right hip fracture with open reduction, internal fixation.

10. Active range of motion bilateral lower extremities within functional limits.

11. Patient instructed in use of transcutaneous electrical nerve stimulator, on an as-needed basis.

12. Chest physical therapy performed for 20 minutes, percussion and vibration to right lower lobe.

13. Patient was discharged from the neonatal intensive care unit on 3/3/00.

14. Past medical history: insulin-dependent diabetes mellitus for 5 years, high blood pressure for 10 years.

15. Magnetic resonance imaging revealed moderate left middle cerebral artery cerebral vascular accident.

EXERCISE 2-3

1. Pt. underwent CABG 3/17/99; **or** Pt. s/p CABG 3/17/99.

2. PT to coordinate ADL practice with OT and RN staff.

3. Pt.'s HR Δ'd (or ↑'d) from 90 to 120 p̄ 3 min of walking at comfortable speed.

4. Pt.'s OB/GYN reported pt. has experienced LBP t/o pregnancy.

5. Pt.'s daughter reports that pt. has had recent ↓ in fx abilities and h/o falls.

6. BS ↓ B. Pt. instructed in performing DBE b.i.d.

7. Pt.'s wife reports that pt. has h/o chronic LBP × 15 yrs.

8. Pt.'s LTG is to walk using only str. cane.

9. DTR R biceps 2+.

10. Pt. can ↑↓ 1 flight of stairs I, 1 hand on railing.

11. Rx received for PT: ther ex and gait trng.

12. Resident is 82 y.o. and has 1° med dx of CHF.

13. ECG revealed v-tach.

14. Pt. s/p CVA c̄ resultant hemiplegia R UE & LE.

15. HHA instructed to assist pt in AAROM exer, including SLR and hip abd in supine.

CHAPTER 3
EXERCISE 3-1

1. **G**—This sentence states that the child "will" be able to do something; this reflects a goal, and thus belongs in the expected outcomes section.

2. **I**—Limitation in range of motion is a common impairment.

3. **I**—Blood pressure and heart rate also are impairments; they represent the "organ" level of impairments.

4. **R**—A seizure represents a pathologic condition (damage to the cellular process or homeostasis); thus it belongs in Reason for Referral, where pathologic information is listed.

5. **IP**—Patient education is an important component of an Intervention Plan.

6. **R**—Describing a patient's work status or occupation information is a component of his or disability and is listed in Reason for Referral.

7. **F**—Stair climbing is a functional skill.

8. **A**—This statement links impairments (poor expiratory ability) with function (ineffective cough and lowered endurance for daily care activities). The linkage provides the foundation for a PT diagnosis and is stated in the Assessment section of a report.

9. **R**—Describing a patient's profession or occupation is listed in Reason for Referral.

10. **G**—This sentence states that the patient "will" be able to stand at the bathroom sink; this reflects a goal and thus belongs in the expected outcomes section.

11. **IP**—Therapeutic exercise is a commonly used intervention by physical therapists.

12. **I**—Muscle strength is a measure of impairments.

13. **A**—This statement links impairments (ineffective right toe clearance; weak R hip musculature) with function (slow and unsafe ambulation indoors). The linkage provides the foundation for a PT diagnosis and is stated in the Assessment section of a report.

14. **F**—Lifting a box is a functional skill.

15. **IP**—Coordinating intervention with other professionals (OT and nursing staff) is documented in the Intervention Plan.

CHAPTER 4

EXERCISE 4-1

Example	What is Wrong?	Rewrite Statement (Examples)
1. Pt. had surgery yesterday.	Time course and type of surgery (related to disease process) is not specified. Best to indicate date of surgery rather than "yesterday"	*Pt. underwent L total hip replacement (posterior approach) 7/2/98.*
2. Pt. reports pain.	Type of pain and location is not described in detail; does not provide meaningful information about the pathologic condition.	*Pt. reports pain in central low back, radiating into left buttock, which began 2 wks ago.*
3. Pt. is a young male amputee.	Not enough detail. Location and type of amputation is not included. *Young* is a vague descriptor; age of patient should be specified. Statement is labeling; people-first terminology is not used.	*Pt. is an 18-year-old male with a right transtibial amputation.*
4. Pt. had a right-sided stroke.	Location and time course of stroke is not specified.	*Pt. had a R MCA stroke on 12/5/01.*
5. Kelly's mother reports that there is family history of hip problems.	Not enough detail. Type of hip problem is not indicated. This statement would only be included if it is relevant to a patient's problems.	*Kelly's mother reports that there is a family history of hip dislocations similar to Kelly's.*
6. Pt. is taking multiple medications for various medical problems.	Not enough detail; names of medications should be included, and for which conditions when known.	*Pt. is currently taking 2.0 mg Haldol daily to minimize involuntary movements; 20 mg Paxil for depression.*
7. Pt. has amyotrophic lateral sclerosis.	Time course not specified. In many brain diseases, such as amyotrophic lateral sclerosis, the type of pathology and location are generally encompassed within the disease name; depending on the audience, more information could be provided.	*Pt. was diagnosed with amyotrophic lateral sclerosis, a degenerative disease affecting upper and lower motor neurons, 18 months ago.*
8. Pt. has typical problems related to aging.	"Typical problems" has a negative connotation and does not have enough detail. The specific problems the patient is experiencing should be described.	*Pt. reports general forgetfulness of short-term events but does not report any problems with long-term memory.*
9. Pt. is taking anti-spasticity meds.	Not enough detail. *Anti-spasticity* is a general term that could apply to several different drugs.	*Pt. is currently taking Baclofen to reduce spasticity.*
10. Pt. has a family hx of heart problems.	Not enough detail. *Heart problems* is a very broad term. Providing information about the type of heart problems might be important.	*Pt. has family history of coronary artery disease.*
11. Pt. complains of fatigue.	Type of fatigue and time course not specified. "Complains of" has a negative connotation and should be avoided.	*Pt.'s primary problem is general fatigue, which has been constant for the past 3 wks, and does not change based on activity level or time of day.*
12. Referring physician reports that pt. may need to have surgery.	Not enough detail; physician's name and specific type of surgery are not included.	*The referring physician, Dr. Rothman, stated that pt. might require a L4-5 laminectomy.*

Example	What is Wrong?	Rewrite Statement (Examples)
13. Pt. has a broken leg	Location, time course, and type of fracture is not specified.	*Pt. fractured his R femur (comminuted) on 1/23/02.*
14. Pt. has cancer.	Type of cancer and time course of condition are not specified.	*Pt. was diagnosed with colon cancer on 8/2/00 and is currently receiving chemotherapy.*
15. Jenny's mother reports that she began crawling and walking late.	Not enough detail. This statement is typically part of a developmental history for a young child. The exact age at which the child began crawling and walking would be important to include.	*Jenny began crawling at 12 mon and walking at 20 mon.*

EXERCISE 4-2

Background Information:
(10) Chelsea is a 12 y.o. girl in the 7th grade who attends Jonesbridge Middle School. (7) Chelsea was referred by the Smithtown School District for this independent PT evaluation to assist in educational planning.

Current Condition:
(11) Chelsea has a diagnosis of myotonic dystrophy, a form of muscular dystrophy resulting in muscle weakness and accompanied by myotonia (delayed relaxation of muscles after contraction). (3) Chelsea first began showing symptoms of myotonic dystrophy when she was in 3rd grade. (12) Chelsea's primary concern is that she gets fatigued when walking between classes.

Past Medical History:
(1) Chelsea's mother, Mrs Green, provided background information regarding Chelsea's past medical history. (8) Chelsea has not had any surgeries and has not been hospitalized for any reason.

Medications:
(4) She is not currently taking any medications.

Other (Family History)
(6) There is a history of myotonic dystrophy in Chelsea's family, so Mrs. Green and Chelsea were very familiar with related symptoms and problems.

Statements that Do Not Belong in this Section:
(2) Chelsea has significant weakness in her arms and legs—this is a very vague description of muscle strength. A more specific description of weakness (e.g., manual muscle testing) should be written in the Impairments section.
(5) Chelsea enjoys math and art classes at school—not relevant information for a PT evaluation.
(9) Chelsea is able to ascend and descend a full flight of stairs—this belongs in the Functional Abilities section because it describes performance in a specific functional skill.

CHAPTER 5

EXERCISE 5-1

Statement	What is Wrong?	Rewrite Statement
1. Able to walk 50 feet with straight cane.	Inappropriate for this section. Measures function, not disability. This statement provides detailed information about functional abilities. Disability would address global abilities.	*Before injury, pt. was able to walk I s̄ AD.*
2. Needs help with some activities.	Not enough detail. Describe general type of activities.	*Pt. needs A of HHA for some ADLs.*
3. Pt. is a T12 paraplegic who is confined to a wheelchair.	Inappropriate for this section. Information about medical diagnosis (T12 paraplegia) belongs in the Reason for Referral: background information section. Also, statement is labeling; not written in people-first language. Refer to patient as "a patient with T12 paraplegia." *Confined to a wheelchair* also has a negative connotation.	*Pt. uses a lightweight W/C with gel seat cushion for primary means of indoor and outdoor mobility.*
4. Has poor motivation to return to work.	*Poor motivation* has a negative connotation and reflects your opinion rather than an objective finding. Stick to objective findings about patient's participation in rehabilitation program.	*Pt. reports that he is not interested in returning to work.*
5. Works on a loading dock.	Not enough detail. Pt.'s general responsibilities and level of physical activity requirement on the job need to be identified.	*Pt. works on a loading dock lifting boxes as heavy as 50 lbs, up to 8 hr/day.*
6. TBI pt. requires A c̄ all ADLs.	Does not use person-first language. Eliminate *TBI pt.* and refer to just "pt." Including specific caregivers is useful.	*Pt. requires A c̄ all ADLs from nursing staff.*
7. Pt. enjoys outdoor sports.	Not enough detail. Include specific sports and level of participation.	*Client enjoys hiking 1-2 × month and skiing 10-12 × during winter months.*
8. Pt. complains that she cannot return to work 2° to architectural barriers.	Negative connotation. Avoid word *complains.* Architectural barriers not specifically defined.	*Pt. reports that 8 stairs in front entrance of office building limit her ability to enter the building and thus return to work.*
9. Pt. will return to work in full capacity in 8 weeks.	Inappropriate for this section. This is a goal not a disability statement.	*Pt. is currently unable to work as a carpenter 2° to inability to lift objects >10 lbs.*
10. Pt. was very active before her injury.	*Very active* does not provide enough detail. Specify type of activity pt. was involved in.	*Pt. led a very active lifestyle before her injury—she bicycled 15 miles 3 × wk and played tennis for 1 hr. 2 × wk.*
11. Suzie's mother reports she doesn't go on any play dates.	Not enough detail. This statement should include information about what is limiting her interactions; otherwise may not be relevant.	*Suzie's mother limits play dates with other children because she feels it can be too overwhelming for Suzie.*

Statement	What is Wrong?	Rewrite Statement
12. Pt. is in poor shape.	Negative connotation; not enough detail.	*Pt. reports he led a relatively inactive lifestyle and has not participated in a regular exercise routine over the past 5 years.*
13. Pt. lives in an apartment.	Important to include whether there are stairs to enter, or stairs within the house, and with whom pt. lives.	*Pt. lives alone on 4th floor of an apartment building, with elevator.*
14. Pt. has a history of bad health habits.	*Bad* does not provide enough detail. Term is too general and not objective.	*Pt. has a history of smoking 2 packs of cigarettes/day for past 30 yrs.*
15. Pt. uses adaptive equipment.	*Adaptive* equipment does not provide enough detail; type of equipment should be specified.	*Pt. uses a raised toilet seat and a shower chair with hand-held shower.*

EXERCISE 5-2

Disability/Social History Documentation

Home Environment: *(2) Pt. lives with her daughter in an apartment building on the 2nd floor. There is an elevator that sometimes doesn't work. (3) Pt. has a raised toilet seat, grab bars, and shower chair in shower. (4) Pt. needs assistance from daughter every other morning for bathing.*

Occupation/Work: *(10) Before surgery, pt. was working 3 days/wk as a retail sales clerk, which required standing and walking most of the day. (7) Pt. is not currently working 2° to walking and standing limitations.*

Health/Occupation Status: *(8) Before surgery, pt. enjoyed 2-3 outings per week to mall or to visit friends. (12) Pt. reports leading a relatively sedentary lifestyle and does not participate in regular exercise program.*

Statements that Do Not Belong in this Section

(1) Pt. underwent L transtibial amputation on 6/18/99 at County Hospital and is now referred for physical therapy evaluation. This statement is related to medical diagnosis and therefore belongs in Medical Diagnosis/History section.

(5) Pt. is able to dress her upper body with setup but requires increased time, verbal cues, and some help to do pants and shoes. Dressing is a functional skill and thus should be documented in Functional Status.

(6) Pt. enjoys watching Jeopardy and Wheel of Fortune every evening. Although this information is related to a person's social/recreational life, the detailed information is not relevant for physical therapy documentation.

(9) Pt. will be independent in outdoor ambulation for distances >1000 ft without assistive device. This documents a functional goal, not a disability statement about current activity level.

(11) Has a hx of IDDM × 10 yrs; HTN × 5 yrs. This statement is also related to medical diagnosis and belongs in Medical History section.

EXERCISE 5-3

CASE REPORT A
Setting: Outpatient

Name: Terry O'Connor   *D.O.B.:* 3/23/33   *Date of Eval:* 7/2/99

Reason For Referral
Current Condition: Right hip bursitis, onset around 5/10/99. Pt. is a 66 y.o. female who had a gradual onset of pain approximately 2 months ago in her right thigh, which progressed to a continuous "burning pain." Pain radiates from the right hip to the right knee. Pt. does not attribute it to any particular incident.

Home Environment: Pt. lives with husband in a 2-story house, 5 steps to enter, with bedroom on 2nd floor.

Occupation/Work: Pt. is retired secretary. Volunteers 1 day/wk at the local hospital but has not volunteered since late May, 2° to pain.

Health Status: Pt. reports that husband has recently been assisting with laundry and household cleaning, which patient previously performed independently. Sleep is frequently disturbed 1-2 ×/night, especially after rolling onto R side, and has difficulty falling asleep due to the pain.

Pt. enjoys cooking and golfing. Doctor advised her to discontinue playing golf until pain subsides. Pt. enjoys playing bridge with her friends once/wk. She is still able to do this but has to modify her position (change from sitting to standing approximately every 10 min). Goes out to lunch or dinner 2-3 ×/week with husband or friends; quality of this activity reduced due to constant position changes.

EXERCISE 5-3

CASE REPORT B
Setting: Inpatient Rehabilitation

Name: Tommy Jones   *D.O.B.:* 5/12/79   *Date of Eval:* 7/2/99   *Admission date:* 7/2/99

Reason For Referral
Current Condition: C7 incomplete SCI 2° to MVA on 6/15/99. Pt. was transferred this morning from County Acute Care Hospital, where he has been since his accident. Medical records reveal one episode of orthostatic hypotension upon coming to sitting and two episodes of autonomic dysreflexia. Pt. underwent surgery on 6/16/99 for anterior cervical fusion. Currently cleared for all rehabilitation activities per Dr. Johnston (per phone conversation this morning).

Home Environment: Before hospital admission, pt. lived at home with his parents while attending college full-time. His parents are very supportive, and his mother is able to stay home to assist with pt.'s care if needed.

Occupation/Work: Pt was full-time engineering student on a large campus. He drove to school and walked long distances (10-15 minutes) between classes. Worked part-time at a local pub as a bartender 2 nights per week.

Health Status: Before injury, household responsibilities included laundry, cleaning room, and mowing lawn weekly. Pt. enjoyed running (completed several marathons), biking, and hiking. Very busy social life in college and with family. Enjoyed going out to dinner and to pubs and to friends' homes. Described health as "good" before injury.

EXERCISE 6-1

Statement	What is Wrong?	Rewrite Statement
1. Able to walk 50 ft.	Context not specified; not enough detail. Describe where pt. can walk, such as surface conditions or specific environment. Also should indicate level of assistance and assistive devices, if applicable.	*Pt. can walk a maximum of 50 ft I'ly, using str cane in hospital corridor; limited due to fatigue.*
2. Able to eat with a spoon with occasional assistance.	*Occasional assistance* is not measurable.	*Able to eat c̄ a spoon c̄ A required 25% of time to prevent spilling.*
3. Pt. is confined to using a wheelchair for long-distance mobility.	*Confined* has a negative connotation; *long-distance mobility* is not measurable.	*Pt. uses a W/C for long distance mobility (>500 ft) outside home.*
4. Able to climb a few stairs.	Not enough detail. Provide more details on capability. *A few* is not measurable Indicate # of stairs, pattern of stair climbing or speed	*Pt. can ↑↓ 10 steps, step-over-step, c̄ 1 hand on R↑ railing.*
5. Can throw a ball but cannot catch one.	Not enough detail; not measurable. Describe size of ball, distance thrown.	*Can throw an 8-inch ball 5 ft 3/4 trials; unable to catch from 3 ft distance 0/4 trials*
6. Can walk on uneven surfaces.	The term *uneven surfaces* is not sufficiently detailed; not measurable.	*Pt. can walk outdoors on grass I'ly.*
7. Pt. is not motivated to walk.	*Not motivated* has a negative connotation and is an interpretation by the therapist, not an objective statement.	*Pt. would not attempt ambulation. Pt. reports he is not yet "ready to try to walk," despite advice by PT and MD that he is medically ready.*
8. Dresses upper body with difficulty.	*Difficulty* not measurable; specify degree of difficulty—which components of dressing are problematic?	*Pt. needs min A to get arms through shirts and to do most buttons.*
9. Walks slowly.	Not enough detail; not measurable; context not specified. Provide speed of ambulation to provide measurable data.	*Pt.'s avg walking speed on indoor level surface is 60 m/min (avg. for an adult her age is 90 m/min).*
10. Pt. doesn't drive.	Not enough detail; specify why the patient does not drive.	*Pt. does not drive >20 min at a time 2° to pain in neck and R arm.*
11. C/o pain during standing.	Focus should be on standing (a Function) not on pain (an Impairment). *Complains of* has a negative connotation. Also not measurable—specify time the patient can stand and where the pain is.	*Pt. is able to stand for max. 15 min. After this, pt. reports gradual increase in LBP (rated up to 4/10 on VAS), and needs to sit after 20-25 min.*
12. Transfers with assistance.	*Assistance* is not measurable; not enough detail; specify how much assistance is required and the type of transfer.	*Transfers from bed → W/C c̄ max A using a stand-pivot transfer.*
13. Pt. can lift various size boxes.	Not measurable; provide more information about boxes (e.g., weight), and also to what height boxes can be lifted.	*Pt. can lift boxes up to 10 lbs from floor to waist-height shelf.*
14. Pt. can't get up from a low chair.	Not measurable; quantify amount of assistance needed and height of chair.	*Pt. needs min A to rise to stand from 16-inch height chair.*
15. Pt. is having trouble sitting for extended periods at work.	Not measurable; quantify how long pt. can sit for, and specify why he cannot sit longer.	*Pt. unable to sit at work desk for >20 min at a time 2° to back pain.*

EXERCISE 6-2

FUNCTIONAL STATUS DOCUMENTATION

Ambulation
(3) Pt. walks 200 ft in hospital hallway c̄ supervision c̄↑ in HR to 120 bpm.

Stairs and Curbs
(5) Pt. can ↑↓ 10 stairs with 1 railing, step over step, in 22 sec.
(11) Pt. can ↑↓ 6" and 8" curbs c̄ CG.

ADLs
(4) Pt. performs daily morning routine of brushing teeth and shaving in 5 min s̄ SOB while standing. (13) Able to dress upper body I'ly; requires mod A to reach down to put on pants and don shoes and socks from a seated position.

Transfers
(8) Pt. transfers from bed to W/C c̄ supervision.

STATEMENTS THAT DO NOT BELONG IN FUNCTIONAL STATUS SECTION
(1) Pt. will return to work in 4 wks. This statement reflects a goal at the disability level.
(2) Pt. is s/p CABG × 4. This is a medical diagnosis stating that the patient recently underwent heart surgery.
(6) Strength B knee extension 4/5. Strength is an impairment. This statement belongs in the Impairment section.
(7) Pt. has 20 yr. history of IDDM. Information about a patient's medical history belongs in reasons for referral section (past medical history).
(9) B ankle pitting edema c̄ circumferential measurement L>R by 0.75". This measure of edema reflects an impairment—loss or abnormality at the tissue or body system level.
(10) PROM B LE WFL x̄ B ankle DF to 0°. Limitations in passive range of motion are impairments.
(12) Pt. performed ADLs I prior to surgery. This statement documents the patient's prior functional status. Such statements are typically listed in Disability and Social History section (Health Status).

EXERCISE 6-3

Bus Driver
Sitting
Turning wheel
Operating door
Shifting gears
Walking up and down stairs
Walking (approx. 50 ft)
Turning head to look behind both ways

Homemaker
Cooking—carrying pots and pans, standing to cook
Cleaning—mopping, vacuuming, washing dishes
Laundry
Financial management
Shopping (walking, pushing cart, reaching to shelves, carrying groceries)

College Student
Sitting
Reading/turning pages
Traveling to and from classes
Traveling up and down stairs

Administrative Assistant
Typing
Filing
Computer skills
Sitting
Walking

Professional Basketball Player
Dribbling
Free throw
Running
Blocking
Jumping
Passing
Shooting
Walking backwards and sideways

CHAPTER 7

EXERCISE 7-1

Impairment Statement	Impairment Category
1. R elbow flexion PROM 0-60°.	Range of motion
2. Walks with uneven step lengths and ↑ weight-bearing time on R side.	Gait, locomotion, and balance
3. Sensation intact B LEs below knee 10/10 correct responses.	Sensory integrity
4. Mini-Mental State Examination score 19/30.	Arousal, attention, and cognition
5. AROM B UEs WFL.	Range of motion
6. Right facial nerve intact.	Cranial and peripheral nerve integrity
7. Circumference mid-patella L knee: 10"; R knee: 9.25".	Anthropometric characteristics
8. Rates pain in low back as 5/10 on VAS after sitting for 10 min; pain described as aching/throbbing.	Pain
9. Skin intact B LE and trunk.	Integumentary integrity
10. Berg balance scale score = 31/56 indicating high risk for falls.	Gait, locomotion, and balance
11. Demonstrates antalgic gait pattern.	Gait, locomotion, and balance
12. B patellar tendon reflexes 2+/5.	Reflex integrity
13. B lung fields clear to auscultation.	Aerobic capacity/endurance ventilation AND and respiration/gas exchange
14. Incentive spirometry in sitting $\bar{c}$ maximal volume = 1750 ml.	Aerobic capacity/endurance ventilation AND and respiration/gas exchange
15. Pt. has forward head and flattened lumbar lordosis.	Posture
16. Pt. is alert and oriented to × 2 (person and place).	Arousal, attention, and cognition
17. HR ↑'d to 110 beats/min $\bar{p}$ 5 minutes of walking at 1.0 m/sec.	Aerobic capacity/endurance
18. Proprioception sensation impaired L ankle 2/8 correct responses.	Sensory integrity

Impairment Statement	Impairment Category
19. R hand grip strength is 15 kg as measured by hand-held dynamometer, avg. 3 trials.	Muscle performance
20. Eye movements, smooth pursuit and visual fields intact (cranial nerves II, III, IV, and VI).	Cranial and peripheral nerve integrity

EXERCISE 7-2

Statement	What is Wrong?	Rewrite Statement
1. Sensation is impaired.	*Impaired* is not measurable. Not enough detail; describe where sensation is impaired; quantify extent of impairment.	*Sensation impaired dorsal aspect R foot, 2/5 correct responses.*
2. ROM is moderately limited.	*Moderately limited* is not measurable; ROM can be measured in degrees. Not enough detail; specify ROM of a specific joint and motion.	*ROM R knee flexion 0-85°.*
3. Pt. c/o excruciating pain.	*Excruciating* is not measurable; describe location, quality, severity, timing, intensity, what makes pain better/worse.	*Pt. reports pain in L shoulder at glenohumeral joint ("stabbing"), onset 3 days ago. Rates pain as 4/10 on VAS in a.m., 8/10 in p.m. Pain is relieved by lying down (2/10)*
4. Pt. walks with L knee pain.	Not measurable; not enough detail. Focus is on "walking" and not on pain. For this statement to belong in the Impairment section, it should focus on the pain specifically. Describe location, quality, severity, timing, and what makes pain better/worse.	*Pt. reports L knee pain began approx. 2 months ago. Pain described as "sharp," located on medial aspect of L knee; pt. rates pain as 3/10 at rest (sitting or lying down), ↑s to 7/10 after walking 5 min.*
5. Pt. has L leg edema.	Not enough detail; specify where the edema is (ankle, calf, knee, etc.). Not measurable; quantify degree of edema.	*2+ pitting edema L ankle; circumference L ankle at malleoli 26 cm, R ankle 22 cm.*
6. Pt. demonstrates a significant ↑ in HR c̄ stair climbing.	*Significant* is not measurable; HR can be measured quantitatively.	*HR increases from 80 to 120 bpm p̄ pt. ↑ 24 steps.*
7. Pt's. reflexes are hyperactive.	Not enough detail; specific reflex not identified. *Hyperactive* is not measurable; reflexes can be quantified.	*Patellar tendon reflex: L 2+; R 3+.*
8. Pt. doesn't know what's going on.	Not appropriate; if pt.'s cognitive status is being documented, not enough detail is provided.	*Pt. is alert and oriented × 3 (person, place, and time).*
9. Pt. has abnormal gait pattern.	*Abnormal* is not measurable; should identify what specifically is not normal.	*Pt. walks c̄ L Trendelenburg gait, indicative of gluteus medius weakness.*
10. Pt. has poor endurance.	*Poor* is not measurable; not specific to an activity, which is important for endurance. Endurance can be measured on a perceived exertion scale.	*Pt. reports SOB (11/15 on BORG) and has HR ↑ to 140 bpm p̄ walking 200 ft.*

EXERCISE 7-3

IMPAIRMENT DOCUMENTATION

Posture

(2) Mild L thoracic C-curve scoliosis.

ROM

(4) PROM limited R ankle DF −5°.

Sensation

(8) Impaired sensation B LE: L4 dermatome 2/5 correct responses on R, 3/5 on L; L5, S1, S2 dermatomes 0/5 correct responses B.

Proprioception

(5) Proprioception impaired B ankle—0/7 correct responses.

Strength

(6) Strength B LEs; hip flexion 5/5 B; hip extension 0/5 B; hip abduction 5/5 B; knee extension R 4/5, L 4+/5; knee flexion R 2+/5, L 3−/5; ankle DF R 2/5, L 2+/5; ankle PF R 0/5, L 1/5.

Anthropometric Measures

(9) Leg length discrepancy 3/4″, R>L.

Systems review

(11) Vision is intact.

Statements that Do Not Belong in Impairment Section

(1) 8 y.o. child with diagnosis of spina bifida. Spina bifida is a medical diagnosis. This information belongs in the Reason for Referral/Current Condition section.

(3) Walks on flat tile surface in hallway 100 feet with B loftstrand crutches in 1 min. Documentation of walking ability (distance, use of assistive device) describes a functional skill. This belongs in the Functional Status section.

(7) Mother will be instructed in home program to improve ankle ROM. Instruction/education to a family member or caregiver is part of the intervention plan. This statement should be documented in the Intervention plan.

(10) Uses W/C for long-distance mobility outside home. General mobility, whether by wheelchair or walking, represents a functional ability. This statement belongs in the Functional Status section.

(12) Strength in R ankle PF will increase to 3/5. This is a statement of a goal written at the impairment level.

CHAPTER 8

EXERCISE 8-1

Medical Diagnosis	Assessment
CASE 1 59 y.o. male, R THR 2° to osteoarthritis, 3 wks previous. Pt. past acute stage—no significant pain or swelling; incision well healed. **Disability** Sales representative, travels by car, unable to work since surgery **Functional limitations** Needs assist for transfers to car, walks slowly with walker, up to 100 ft at a time, needs assist on steps **Impairments** Weakness in R hip flexors, abductors, and extensors; habitual gait deviations from pre-op antalgic gait; R hip flexion and abduction ROM limited.	Pt. is a 59 y.o. male, 3 wks s/p R THR 2° to osteoarthritis. Incision is healing well, and pt. experiences no significant pain or swelling. Weakness in hip musculature, hip ROM limitations, and pre-op giat deviations have resulted in limited speed and distance for walking. Weakness also makes transfer in and out of car impossible without assistance. Limitations in walking and car transfers are currently preventing pt. from returning to work as a sales rep. Pt. requires PT intervention to improve strength, ROM, and walking ability, facilitating pt.'s return to work.

Medical Diagnosis	Assessment

CASE 2

43 y.o. female with multiple sclerosis diagnosed 3 yrs previous; recovering from recent exacerbation

Disability

Clerical worker in major downtown office building; rides train and bus to work; resists using cane. Pt. is fearful of falling during commute and needs extra time to commute.

Functional limitations

Requires assist to go up and down steps; walks slowly; walking difficulties exacerbated in crowded places

Impairments

Only mild weakness; standing balance easily disturbed, esp. when pt. is distracted

Pt. is a 43 y.o. female diagnosed c̄ MS 3 years ago. Pt. presents c̄ significantly impaired standing balance, resulting in slowed walking speed and difficulties walking in crowded places and negotiating stairs. These problems are limiting pt.'s ability to safely and efficiently commute to work. Pt. requires PT intervention to address balance and ambulation difficulties and improve ability to commute to work.

CASE 3

39 y.o. female with diagnosis of cervical strain. Onset of symptoms occurred 6 wks ago.

Disability

CPA at local firm, currently unable to tolerate typical 8-10 hr workday secondary to symptoms. Majority of time typically spent on phone and on computer.

Functional limitations

Occasionally requires pain medication to assist with sleeping at night. Unable to talk on phone secondary to pain with phone cradling position. Unable to tolerate computer work >2 hrs secondary to increased pain.

Impairments

Static sitting posture presents with a decrease in cervical lordosis and an increase in thoracic kyphosis. Limited AROM with right-side flexion and rotation and c-spine. Flexed, rotated, and sidebent left at C5 and C6. Weakness in bilateral lower trapezius: 3/5, bilateral middle trapezius/rhomboids: 4/5, and cervical extensors: 3+/5. Pain rated as 3/10 at rest and 6/10 after working 2 hrs; described as throbbing and occasionally "shooting."

Pt. is a 39 y.o. female with recent diagnosis of cervical strain; onset of symptoms 6 weeks ago. Pt. presents with poor cervical and thoracic postures, moderate ROM and strength deficits in the cervical and thoracic spine regions, cervical facet dysfunction, and increased pain that results in limited tolerance with computer and phone duties, as well as sleep disturbance. These issues are restricting the pt.'s work endurance and performance. Pt. requires PT to address postural dysfunction, ROM, and strength deficits, as well as facet dysfunction. Postural education, proper body mechanics, ergonomic assessment, and pain management would be addressed as well.

CHAPTER 9

EXERCISE 9-1

1. Independent in transfers in 2 wks.
   Patient (A) will transfer (B) independently (D) between bed and wheelchair (C) with 100% success rate (D) within 2 wks (E).

   Type: Functional

   Problem: A, B, C

2. Pt. will be functional in ADL within 3 wks.
   Patient (A) will perform (B) all ADLs (C) independently (D) within 3 wks (E).

   Type: Disability

   Problem: B, C, D

3. Return to work in 3 months.
   Patient (A) will return (B) to work as kindergarten teacher (C) and be able to participate (B) in all required activities (C) within 3 months (E).

   Type: Disability

   Problem: A, C, D

4. Increased strength in quadriceps to 5/5 bilaterally.
   Strength in B quadriceps (C) will increase (B) to 5/5 (D) within 3 wks (E).

   NOTE: *Actor is typically not specified for Impairment goal.*

   Type: *Impairment*

   Problem: B, E

5. Pt. will ↑↓ stairs in 1 min.
   Pt. (A) will ↑↓ (B) 1 flight/12 steps (C) at 7" height (C) c̄ 1 rail (C) using step-over-step pattern (D) in 1 minute (D) I'ly (D) within 3 wks (E).

   Type: Functional

   Problem: C, E

6. *Pt. will demonstrate increased R hip ROM.*
   AROM R hip flexion (C) will increase (B) to 110° (D) in 2 wks (E).

   Type: *Impairment*

   Problem: C, D, E

7. Pt. will return to school.
   Pt. (A) will return (B) to college (C) taking 2 classes (D) within 1 month (E).

   Type: *Disability*

   Problem: C, D, E

8. Maintain upright posture while sitting.
    Pt. (A) will be able to maintain (B) upright sitting posture in W/C (C) for 2 hrs (D) s̄ hypotensive episode (D) within 1 wk (E).

    Type: *Impairment*

    Problem: A, C, D, E

9. Pt. will get from his room to therapy.
    Pt. (A) will propel his W/C (B) from his room to therapy gym (approx. 250 ft) (C) in less than 3 min (D) within 2 weeks (E).

    Type: *Functional*

    Problem: B, D, E

10. Pt. will perform 10 reps of straight leg raises.
    Strength R hip flexors (C) will increase (B) to 3+/5 (D) within 2 weeks (E).

    or

    Pt. (A) will perform (B) 10 reps (D) of straight leg raises on mat as part of exercise routine (C) within 2 wks (E).

    Type: *Impairment*

    Problem: C, E

EXERCISE 9-2

Statement	What is Wrong?	Rewrite Statement
1. Pt. will experience less pain.	Reports of pain are related to impairment goals. Focus should be on task or function. *Less pain* is not measurable. Where is the pain, during what activity?	*Pt. will walk >500 ft distance c̄ pain <4/10 on VAS, 4/5 days within 2 wks.*
2. Pt. will progress from a walker to a cane within 3 wks.	Not enough detail regarding distance or context. Progress will be obvious when all notes are reviewed. Reflects the process rather than the goal.	*Pt. will walk 100 ft on level surfaces using a straight cane c̄ CS in 3 wks.*
3. Educate pt. on hip precautions within 2 sessions.	Educating the pt. is part of the intervention, not a goal. Reflects the process rather than the goal.	*Pt. will verbally demonstrate knowledge of total hip precautions when asked by therapist 100% of the time.*
4. Return to work.	Not concrete re: specific work requirements and situation. Not measurable.	*Pt. will sit at desk at work 30 min at a time c̄ pain < 2/10 on VAS within 3 wks.*
5. Pt. will walk with a normal gait pattern within 4 wks.	Not measurable. *Normal* is a relative term and depends upon their status prior to recent injury.	*Pt. will amb. 500 ft s̄ an assistive device, in the hospital hallways, c̄ CG in 3 wks.*
6. Pt. will walk independently with a quad cane for distances up to 500 ft within 3 wks.	This is a good example of a functional goal; only the context is missing.	*Pt. will walk independently with a quad cane for distances up to 500 ft on tiled surfaces within 3 wks.*

Statement	What is Wrong?	Rewrite Statement
7. Pt. will be I in all activities in 2 wks.	Not enough detail; *all activities* is too vague.	*Pt. will transfer independently from W/C to the toilet using a SB in < 1 min in 2 wks.*
8. Pt. will ascend and descend stairs within 3 days.	Not concrete; not enough detail. Height of stairs, time to complete, use of railing can all be used to clarify goal.	*Pt. will ascend/descend 12 8" height steps, using step over step pattern, within 30 sec, within 5 days.*
9. Pt. will not have pain when reaching.	Emphasis is on pain, which relates to impairments; not enough detail describing functional skill of reaching.	*Pt. will put away dishes from dishwasher to all shelves without report of pain (0/10 on VAS), within 1 wk.*
10. Strength R knee / will increase to 4/5 within 3 wks.	This is a well-written Impairment goal—not appropriate when writing Functional goals. A Functional goal would utilize a task in which knee / strength is critical.	*Pt. will ↑ 10 steps SOS s̄ railing in 3 wks.*

CHAPTER 10

EXERCISE 10-1

Statement	What is Wrong?	Rewrite Statement
1. Practice walking.	Not enough detail. Where will the patient be walking? Describe circumstances, type of walking; no indication of skilled services required.	*Gait training—practice walking within home from bedroom to bathroom, living room, and kitchen to address safety and teach compensatory strategies for visual field deficits and L spatial neglect.*
2. Apply hot-packs.	Rationale not provided; not enough detail. Why is a hot-pack needed? Specify to address pain, relax tissues, etc. Area of body needs to be stated. No indication of skilled services required.	*Moist heat to cervical spine to promote relaxation and improve cervical spine flexibility.*
3. Pt. will be able to walk 10 ft to the bathroom.	Not appropriate for this section. This is a goal not an intervention. Need to state it in terms of what the pt. or therapist will do.	*Practice walking for short distances to bathroom, using manual guidance as needed to improve foot clearance.*
4. Pt. will be given strengthening exercises.	Not enough detail. Describe what type of strengthening exercises. Be specific to muscle group. *Instructed* is a better term than given.	*Pt. will be instructed in home program to include isometric strengthening for left quadriceps.*
5. Coordinate care with all nursing personnel.	Not enough detail. What care will be coordinated? Clarify the PT-related activities you will coordinate with nurses on—transfers, bed mobility, etc.	*Will review transfers and bed mobility strategies, which will most effectively facilitate pt.'s use of right side of body with nursing aides.*

Statement	What is Wrong?	Rewrite Statement
6. Assess work environment.	Not enough detail. This could involve many different things; try to clarify which areas of the work environment will be addressed. What is the purpose of assessing work environment?	*Work environment to be assessed within 2 weeks to make modification recommendations prior to returning to work.*
7. Pt. will increase right hamstring strength.	Not appropriate for this section. This is a goal not an intervention. Need to state this as what the patient or therapist will do.	*Progressive resistive strengthening exercises for R hamstrings.*
8. Balance training.	Not enough detail. Need to identify what specifically will be addressed with this training.	*Training of sitting balance including proactive (reaching, ball play activities) and reactive (response to perturbations in sitting, activities on therapeutic ball) to improve overall sitting ability.*
9. Pt. will receive ultrasound at 1.0 W/cm², 1 MHz to R quadriceps (VMO), in a 10 cm area just proximal and slightly medial to right knee, moving ultrasound head slowly in circular fashion for 10 min, each session.	Too much detail is provided. It would be sufficient to eliminate some of the details; parameters could be specified in daily notes. Rationale for the intervention is not stated.	*Pt. will receive ultrasound to R quadriceps (VMO) in order to improve mobility and promote tissue healing.*
10. Pt. will take pain relief medication as needed.	Not appropriate for this section. Prescribing or recommending medication is not within the scope of physical therapy practice. This information should not be included in this section of the report, and might only be included in the Medical Diagnosis section.	*Move to Diagnosis section and restate: Pt. reports taking pain relief medication prescribed by his primary care physician as needed to reduce back pain.*
11. Home evaluation.	Not enough detail; rationale for doing a home evaluation not provided.	*Home evaluation will be conducted prior to D/C to evaluate pt.'s home environment and accessibility*
12. Reduce R ankle edema.	Not appropriate for this section. This is a general goal, not an intervention. The method used to reduce the edema would be appropriate to document in the intervention section	*Ice to be applied to R ankle to ↓ swelling and pain.*
13. Teach family to care for patient.	Not enough detail; document specific skills being taught	*Educate pt.'s family members on safe techniques for W/C transfers ↔ car and bed.*
14. Practice pressure-relief techniques.	Not enough detail; not specific as to type of pressure relief.	*Educate pt. in effective pressure-relief techniques while sitting in W/C to prevent skin breakdown.*
15. E-stim to anterior tibialis.	Rationale not provided	*E-stim to anterior tibialis for muscle re-education.*

EXERCISE 10-2

INTERVENTION PLAN

(8) Pt. will be seen 3×/wk for outpatient physical therapy, 45-min sessions.

Coordination/Communication

(3) Referral to orthotist to evaluate for specific AFO.
(7) Discuss with patient options for long distance mobility, including use of wheelchair.

Patient-Related Instruction

(2) Pt. will be instructed in self-stretching of right wrist and elbow.
(11) Pt. will view video-modeling strategies for improved UE function in patients who have had a stroke.
(13) Pt. will be instructed in home walking program to improve speed and endurance; walking daily beginning with 10 min and progressing to 20 min over 4 wks.

Procedural Interventions

(5) Fx training to address balance and coordination during morning bathroom routine.
(10) Trng with appropriate assistive device (straight cane or quad cane) during ambulation indoors and outdoors and transfers to improve safety, speed and distance.
(6) RLE strengthening exercises such as squats, stair stepping, and obstacle negotiation to improve standing and walking ability.

Statements that Do Not Belong in this Section

(1) Medical hx is significant for HTN. This statement belongs in Reason for Referral: Medical/Surgical History.
(4) Pt. will be able to negotiate walking over 6-inch high obstacles. This is a statement of a functional goal-belongs in Goals section.
(9) Strength of right hip abductors will increase to 4/5. This is a statement of an impairment goal—belongs in Goals section.
(12) Pt. can ↑↓ 10 steps in 1 min 20 sec. This statement of a function—belongs in Functional Status section.

CHAPTER 11

EXERCISE 11-1

SOAP Statement	SOAP Section G, S, O, A, P
1. Performed 10 reps SLR B.	O
2. Pt. reports she was able to walk with her daughter out to get the mail yesterday and did not experience any dizziness.	S
3. Treatment next session will include progression to stationary bike × 10 min.	P
4. Pt. walked 15 ft from bed to bathroom without SOB, in 30 sec.	O
5. Pt. states that she "felt sore" after last treatment session.	S
6. Pt. is progressing well with increasing repetitions of LE strengthening exercises and has achieved goal #1.	A
7. Pitting edema noted in R ankle.	O
8. Pt. was instructed to continue to maintain R leg in elevated position while sitting at desk during the day.	O
9. Pt. will transfer from bed to wheelchair independently, 4/5 trials within 2 wks.	A
10. Pt. states she is anxious to return to work.	S
11. Pt. will continue with daily walking program at home during off-therapy days, progressing to 20 min each day by next wk.	P

SOAP Statement	SOAP Section G, S, O, A, P
12. Pt. will stand c̄ A for up to 1 min within 1 wk.	P
13. Pt. reports pain in low back while walking as 5/10 on VAS and 8/10 while sitting at desk at work.	S
14. Pt.'s fear of falling is limiting his progress in improving his ability to ambulate in crowded environments and outdoors.	A
15. Pt. reports that she is going back to work on a trial basis next week.	S

EXERCISE 11-2

Statement	Section	What's wrong	Rewrite
1. Pt. states he hates using his walker.	*Subjective*	Not enough detail. It would be helpful to know why he dislikes using his walker.	*Pt. states that he "prefers to use a cane rather than a walker" because it is too difficult to carry things while using the walker.*
2. Pt. says she is so much happier with the care she is receiving at this facility. She was disgusted with her previous medical care; she feels the doctors and therapists were completely noncaring and didn't know what they were doing.	*Subjective*	Too much detail/not appropriate; unnecessary disparagement of other professionals.	*Pt. expressed a desire to seek new professional opinions regarding diagnosis and treatment of her pain.*
3. Pt. has an awkward gait.	*Objective*	Not enough detail; *awkward* is not measurable.	*Pt. walks on indoor level surfaces without A device demonstrates decreased stance time on R 2° to pain in R foot on weight-bearing.*
4. PROM at the R knee is improving.	*Objective*	Not enough detail; not measurable.	*PROM of R knee ✓ is now 0–95°.*
5. Pt. is very confused.	*Objective*	Not enough detail. What is pt. confused about? If performing a mental-status assessment, report findings in an objective manner.	*Pt. is alert & oriented × 1 (person). Mini-mental state examination score: 16/30.*
6. Pt. reports that his son is concerned.	*Subjective*	Not enough detail. Need to document son's specific concerns.	*Pt. reports that his son is concerned about his ability to care for his father when he returns home. Son has a full-time job and 2 small children of his own.*
7. Pt. c/o fatigue after walking for 5 min.	*Subjective*	*Complains of* has a negative connotation.	*Pt. reports feeling fatigued after walking 5 min.*

Statement	Section	What's wrong	Rewrite
8. Timmy has difficulty keeping his head up for prolonged periods.	*Objective*	Not enough detail; not measurable.	*Timmy sustains head erect for an average of 10 sec in 5 trials when asked to look at a picture taped on the chalkboard.*
9. Pt. complains of pain in left shoulder.	*Subjective*	*Complains of* has a negative connotation. Not enough detail.	*Pt. continues to report pain in her L shoulder that radiates down to her elbow, 6/10 on VAS. It aches all of the time except when she is lying down.*
10. Pt. performed 10 reps of knee exercises.	*Objective*	Not enough detail; specific exercises should be documented.	*Pt. performed 10 reps of isometric quad sets.*

EXERCISE 11-3

GOALS

1. (1) ROM B hip flexion will increase to 0-120°
2. (9) Pt. will amb 2000 ft in 6 min independently, negotiating uneven outdoor terrain, HR <110 bpm.
3. (14) Pt. will independently perform transitions stand ⟷ floor.

Subjective (S)

(6) Pt. reports L heel/ankle pain continues; pain at rest in morning 2/10, increases to 5/10 in the afternoon and evening.

Objective (O)

(2) 6-minute walk test—1200′ without assistive device; HR changed from 80 bpm at rest to 120 bpm. (5) Pt. ↑↓ 3 flights (12 stairs) of 8″ steps independently, using SOS pattern to ascend and R rail to descend, SOS; HR ↑ to 120 bpm. (7) Practiced reaching activities in standing, including picking up objects of various weight and height from floor with emphasis on controlled movements and maintaining proper body mechanics. (15) Pt. required min A to transfer from stand to kneeling and kneeling to long sitting. (10) Hip flexion AROM R—0-110°; L—0-95°. (12) Pt. independently performed self-stretching of bilateral gastroc/soleus and hamstrings while sitting on floor; hip flexor stretch in side-lying position (30 sec hold, 3 times each). (11) Inspection of would lateral and posterior aspect of L thigh; reapplied bacitracin, adaptic, and padding to blisters.

Assessment (A)

(4) Pt. has made notable improvement in B hip flexion AROM, which is resulting in improvements in reaching and lifting abilities, and transitions to floor. (13) Pt. continues to improve 6 min walk test and stand ⟷ floor mobility; awaiting x-ray results of L ankle due to pt.'s report of persistent L ankle/heel pain.

Plan (P)

(8) Continue with current Tx plan, with emphasis on soft tissue mobilization, LE flexibility, transitional skills, and improving ambulation and stair climbing ability. (3) Consult with MD this afternoon re: expected x-ray results of L ankle.

Sample Evaluation Forms

Appendix D provides examples of forms that can be used in PT documentation.

Strength & Range of Motion					
Extremities & Trunk:		Strength		ROM	
		Left	Right	Left	Right
Neck	Flexion				
	Extension				
	Rotation				
Shoulder	Flexion 0-180				
	Extension 0-45				
	Abduction 0-180				
	Int Rot 0-70				
	Ext Rot 0-90				
Elbow	Flexion 0-145				
	Extension 0				
Wrist	Flexion 0-80				
	Extension 0-70				
	Fingers				
Trunk	Flexion				
	Extension				
Hip	Flexion 0-125				
	Extension 0-10				
	Abduction 0-45				
	Adduction 0-10				
	Int Rot 0-45				
	Ext Rot 0-45				
Knee	Flexion 0-140				
	Extension 0				
Ankle	Dorsiflex 0-20				
	Plantarflex 0-45				
	Inversion 0-40				
	Eversion 0-20				

FORM A

A sample form used for an examination of strength and ROM. Norm values from Randall, McCreary, Provance (1993).

BODY DIAGRAM

Name:_____ Date:_____

Directions: On the body diagram below, please mark the areas of your symptoms as they are at this moment of your evaluation.

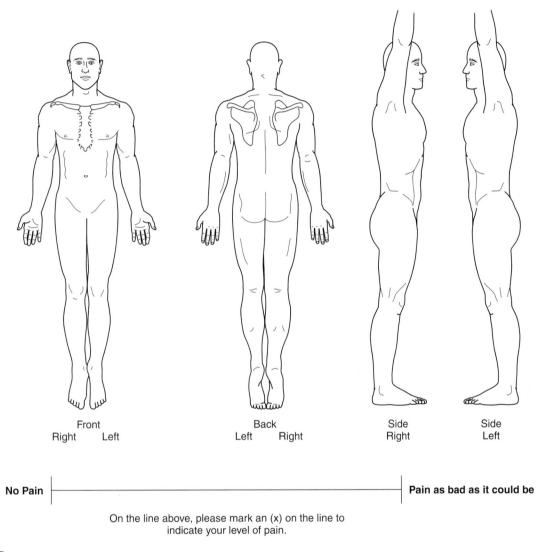

Front	Back	Side	Side
Right Left	Left Right	Right	Left

No Pain ├──┤ **Pain as bad as it could be**

On the line above, please mark an (x) on the line to
indicate your level of pain.

FORM B

A sample pain documentation form. Form is completed by the patient and should be included as part of the medical record.

PHYSICAL THERAPY HOMECARE INITIAL EVALUATION

Name:_____ D.O.B.:_____ Date of Evaluation visit:_____

Address:_____ Phone:_____

Primary MD:_____ Phone:_____

Admitting Diagnosis/date of onset:_____

Past Medical History:_____

_____

Home living situation:_____

Prior functional status:_____

Employment/Recreation/Social Activities:_____

_____

HOME SAFETY ASSESSMENT:

	Safe	Unsafe	Comments/Action taken
1. Kitchen			
2. Bathroom			
3. Living room			
4. Bedroom			
5. Hallways			
6. Stairs in the home			
7. Stairs outside the home			
8. Equiment in the home Specify:_____ _____			
9. Other Specify:_____ _____			

SITTING/STANDING ABILITY *(indicate time & physical limitations, environmental modification and amount of assistance)*

	STATIC	REACTIVE	PROACTIVE
Sitting	☐ Independent	☐ Able to maintain	☐ Able to reach in all directions
	☐ Needs assist	☐ Unable to maintain	☐ Reaching limited
Comments	_____	_____	_____
	_____	_____	_____
Standing	☐ Independent	☐ Able to maintain	☐ Able to reach in all directions
	☐ Needs assist	☐ Unable to maintain	☐ Reaching limited
Comments	_____	_____	_____
	_____	_____	_____

Standardized tests: ☐ Berg Balance Scale_____ ☐ Activities of Balance Confidence_____ ☐ Other:_____

◾ FORM C

A sample evaluation form used in a homecare setting. This form standardizes data collected by therapists, while allowing opportunity for narrative descriptions of patient's functional abilities and impairments.

DAILY LIVING SKILLS

Activity	Assist Code	Comments (strategy, speed, endurance)	Activity	Assist Code	Comments (strategy, speed, endurance)
Bed mobility			Assumes standing position		
Assumes sitting from supine position in bed			Negotiates thresholds		
Lying down in bed from sitting position			Negotiates stairs		
Transfers bed to wheelchair			Bathing		
Transfers to tub			Dressing		
Transfers to toilet			Grooming		
Management of wheelchair			Feeding		
Wheelchair mobility			Housework		
Negotiates doorways			Meal prep		

AMBULATION

Device(s) used:_____

Weight Bearing Status:_____

Assistance needed (see assist code):_____

Distance:_____ time:_____ # steps:_____

Gait:_____

FORM C—cont'd

Continued

IMPAIRMENTS

Passive Range of Motion

Upper:_____

Lower:_____

Trunk & Neck:_____

*Strength/AROM:*_____

_____

Posture: Sitting_____

Standing_____

*Skin Integrity*_____

Sensation   Normal ☐   Abnormal ☐   _____

*Pain:*_____

*Neurological Findings:*_____

Babinski: Positive ☐   Negative ☐   Reflexes:_____

Clonus: Present ☐   Absent   ☐   Muscle tone:_____

Cardiopulmonary/Vital signs: HR_____   BP_____   RR_____   Comments:_____

*Cognitive/mental status:*_____

Other: (include other systems review or pertinent impairments):_____

_____

_____

Patient education/home instructions_____

_____

Patient goals:_____

Patient attitude:_____

Short Range Goals (indicate time frame for each):_____

_____

_____

Long Range Goals (indicate time frame for each):_____

_____

_____

Plan of care:_____

_____

_____

Recommendations:_____

_____

_____   _____

Therapist's name   Therapist's signature

FORM C—cont'd

DEPARTMENT OF HEALTH AND HUMAN SERVICES
HEALTH CARE FINANCING ADMINISTRATION

FORM APPROVED
OMB NO. 0938-0227

PLAN OF TREATMENT FOR OUTPATIENT REHABILITATION (COMPLETE FOR INITIAL CLAIMS ONLY)

1. PATIENT'S LAST NAME	FIRST NAME M.I.	2. PROVIDER NO.	3. HICN
4. PROVIDER NAME	5. MEDICAL RECORD NO. (*Optional*)	6. ONSET DATE	7. SOC. DATE

8. TYPE	9. PRIMARY DIAGNOSIS	10. TREATMENT DIAGNOSIS	11. VISITS FROM SOC.
PT OT SLP CR RT PS SN SW			

12. PLAN OF TREATMENT FUNCTIONAL GOALS   PLAN

GOALS (Short Term)

OUTCOME (*Long Term*)

13. SIGNATURE (*professional establishing POC including prof. designation*)

14. FREQ/DURATION (e.g. 3/Wk x 4 Wk.)

I CERTIFY THE NEED FOR THESE SERVICES FURNISHED UNDER
THIS PLAN OF TREATMENT AND WHILE UNDER MY CARE   ☐ N/A

17. CERTIFICATION
FROM   THROUGH   ☐ N/A

15. PHYSICIAN'S SIGNATURE   16. DATE

18. ON FILE (*Print/type physician's name*)
☐

20. INITIAL ASSESSMENT (*History, medical complications, level of function at
start of care. Reason for referral*)

19. PRIOR HOSPITALIZATION
FROM   THROUGH   ☐ N/A

21. FUNCTIONAL LEVEL (*at end of billing period*) PROGRESS REPORT   ☐ CONTINUE SERVICES OR   ☐ DC SERVICES

22. SERVICE DATES
FROM   THROUGH

FORM HCFA-700 (11-91)

FORM D

Medicare HCFA 700 form for documentation of an initial evaluation and progress report.

DEPARTMENT OF HEALTH AND HUMAN SERVICES
HEALTH CARE FINANCING ADMINISTRATION

FORM APPROVED
OMB NO. 0938-0227

UPDATED PLAN OF PROGRESS FOR OUTPATIENT REHABILITATION
(Complete for Interim to Discharge Claims, Photocopy of HCFA-700 or 701 is required)

1. PATIENT'S LAST NAME	FIRST NAME	M.I.	2. PROVIDER NO.	3. HICN

4. PROVIDER NAME	5. MEDICAL RECORD NO. (*Optional*)	6. ONSET DATE	7. SOC. DATE

8. TYPE PT OT SLP CR	9. PRIMARY DIAGNOSIS	10. TREATMENT DIAGNOSIS	11. VISITS FROM SOC.
RT PS SN SW	12. FREQ/DURATION (e.g. 3/Wk x 4 Wk.)		

13. CURRENT PLAN UPDATE TREATMENT FUNCTIONAL GOALS (*Specifiy changes to goals and plan*)

GOALS (Short Term)

PLAN

OUTCOME (*Long Term*)

I HAVE REVIEWED THIS PLAN OF TREATMENT AND RECERTIFY A CONTINUING NEED FOR SERVICES

15. PHYSICIAN'S SIGNATURE	16. DATE

14. RECERTIFICATION
FROM   THROUGH

17. ON FILE (*Print/type physician's name*)

18. REASON(S) FOR CONTINUING TREATMENT THIS BILLING PERIOD (Clarify goals and necessity for continued skilled care)

19. SIGNATURE (or name of professional, including prof. designation)	20. DATE	21. ☐ CONTINUE SERVICES OR ☐ DC SERVICES

22. FUNCTIONAL LEVEL (at end of billing period - Relate your documentation to functional outcomes and list problems still present)

22. SERVICE DATES
FROM   THROUGH

FORM HCFA-701 (11-91)

FORM E

Medicare HCFA 701 form for documentation of progress and recertification.

INPATIENT REHABILITATION FACILITY - PATIENT ASSESSMENT INSTRUMENT

Identification Information*

1. Facility Information
   A. Facility Name

   _____
   _____
   _____

   B. Facility Medicare
      Provider Number   _____

2. Patient Medicare Number _____

3. Patient Medicaid Number _____

4. Patient First Name _____

5A. Patient Last Name _____

5B. Patient Identification Number _____

6. Birth Date   _____/_____/_____
                        MM / DD / YYYY

7. Social Security Number   _____

8. Gender (1 - Male; 2 - Female)   _____

9. Race/Ethnicity (Check all that apply)
   American Indian or Alaska Native   A. _____
                             Asian   B. _____
             Black or African American   C. _____
                 Hispanic or Latino   D. _____
   Native Hawaiian or Other Pacific Islander   E. _____
                             White   F. _____

10. Marital Status   _____
    (1 - Never Married; 2 - Married; 3 - Widowed;
    4 - Separated; 5 - Divorced)

11. Zip Code of Patient's Pre-Hospital Residence _____

Admission Information*

12. Admission Date   _____/_____/_____
                             MM / DD / YYYY

13. Assessment Reference Date   _____/_____/_____
                                MM / DD / YYYY

14. Admission Class   _____
    (1 - Initial Rehab ; 2 - Evaluation; 3 - Readmission;
    4 - Unplanned Discharge; 5 - Continuing Rehabilitation)

15. Admit From   _____
    (01 - Home; 02 - Board & Care; 03 - Transitional Living;
    04 - Intermediate Care; 05 - Skilled Nursing Facility;
    06 - Acute Unit of Own Facility; 07 - Acute Unit of Another
    Facility; 08 - Chronic Hospital; 09 - Rehabilitation Facility;
    10 - Other; 12 - Alternate Level of Care Unit; 13 – Subacute
    Setting; 14 - Assisted Living Residence)

16. Pre-Hospital Living Setting   _____
    (Use codes from item 15 above)

17. Pre-Hospital Living With   _____
    (Code only if item 16 is 01 - Home;
    Code using 1 - Alone; 2 - Family/Relatives;
    3 - Friends; 4 - Attendant; 5 - Other)

18. Pre-Hospital Vocational Category   _____
    (1 - Employed; 2 - Sheltered; 3 - Student;
    4 - Homemaker; 5 - Not Working; 6 - Retired for
    Age; 7 - Retired for Disability)

19. Pre-Hospital Vocational Effort   _____
    (Code only if item 18 is coded 1 - 4; Code using
    1 - Full-time; 2 - Part-time; 3 - Adjusted Workload)

Payer Information*

20. Payment Source
    A. Primary Source   _____

    B. Secondary Source   _____

    (01 - Blue Cross; 02 - Medicare non-MCO;
    03 - Medicaid non-MCO; 04 - Commercial Insurance;
    05 - MCO HMO; 06 - Workers' Compensation;
    07 - Crippled Children's Services; 08 – Developmental
    Disabilities Services; 09 - State Vocational Rehabilitation;
    10 - Private Pay; 11 - Employee Courtesy;
    12 - Unreimbursed; 13 - CHAMPUS; 14 - Other;
    15 - None; 16 – No-Fault Auto Insurance;
    51 – Medicare MCO; 52 - Medicaid MCO)

Medical Information*

21. Impairment Group   _____   _____
                               Admission   Discharge
    Condition requiring admission to rehabilitation; code
    according to Appendix A, attached.

22. Etiologic Diagnosis   _____
    (Use an ICD-9-CM code to indicate the etiologic problem
    that led to the condition for which the patient is receiving
    rehabilitation)

23. Date of Onset of Impairment   _____/_____/_____
                                  MM / DD / YYYY

24. Comorbid Conditions; Use ICD-9-CM codes to enter up to
    ten medical conditions

    A. _____   B. _____

    C. _____   D. _____

    E. _____   F. _____

    G. _____   H. _____

    I. _____   J. _____

Medical Needs

25. Is patient comatose at admission?   _____
                                           0 - No, 1 - Yes

26. Is patient delirious at admission?   _____
                                           0 - No, 1 - Yes

27. Swallowing Status   _____   _____
                                Admission   Discharge

    3 - *Regular Food:* solids and liquids swallowed safely
         without supervision or modified food consistency
    2 - *Modified Food Consistency/ Supervision:* subject
         requires modified food consistency and/or needs
         supervision for safety
    1 - *Tube /Parenteral Feeding:* tube / parenteral feeding
         used wholly or partially as a means of sustenance

28. Clinical signs of dehydration   _____   _____
                                    Admission   Discharge

    (Code 0 – No; 1 – Yes) e.g., evidence of oliguria, dry
    skin, orthostatic hypotension, somnolence, agitation

*The FIM data set, measurement scale and impairment
codes incorporated or referenced herein are the property of
U B Foundation Activities, Inc. ©1993, 2001 U B Foundation
Activities, Inc. The FIM mark is owned by UBFA, Inc.

OMB-0938-0842 (expires: 01-31-2003)

FORM F

Inpatient Rehabilitation Facility–Patient Assessment Instrument (IRF–PAI).

Continued

INPATIENT REHABILITATION FACILITY - PATIENT ASSESSMENT INSTRUMENT
Page 2

Function Modifiers*

Complete the following specific functional items prior to scoring the FIM™ Instrument:

	ADMISSION	DISCHARGE
29. Bladder Level of Assistance (Score using FIM Levels 1 - 7)	☐	☐
30. Bladder Frequency of Accidents (Score as below)	☐	☐

7 - No accidents
6 - No accidents; uses device such as a catheter
5 - One accident in the past 7 days
4 - Two accidents in the past 7 days
3 - Three accidents in the past 7 days
2 - Four accidents in the past 7 days
1 - Five or more accidents in the past 7 days

Enter in Item 39G (Bladder) the lower (more dependent) score from Items 29 and 30 above.

	ADMISSION	DISCHARGE
31. Bowel Level of Assistance (Score using FIM Levels 1 - 7)	☐	☐
32. Bowel Frequency of Accidents (Score as below)	☐	☐

7 - No accidents
6 - No accidents; uses device such as an ostomy
5 - One accident in the past 7 days
4 - Two accidents in the past 7 days
3 - Three accidents in the past 7 days
2 - Four accidents in the past 7 days
1 - Five or more accidents in the past 7 days

Enter in Item 39H (Bowel) the lower (more dependent) score of Items 31 and 32 above.

	ADMISSION	DISCHARGE
33. Tub Transfer	☐	☐
34. Shower Transfer	☐	☐

(Score Items 33 and 34 using FIM Levels 1 - 7; use 0 if activity does not occur) See training manual for scoring of Item 39K (Tub/Shower Transfer)

	ADMISSION	DISCHARGE
35. Distance Walked	☐	☐
36. Distance Traveled in Wheelchair	☐	☐

(Code items 35 and 36 using: 3 - 150 feet; 2 - 50 to 149 feet; 1 - Less than 50 feet; 0 – activity does not occur)

	ADMISSION	DISCHARGE
37. Walk	☐	☐
38. Wheelchair	☐	☐

(Score Items 37 and 38 using FIM Levels 1 - 7; 0 if activity does not occur) See training manual for scoring of Item 39L (Walk/Wheelchair)

*The FIM data set, measurement scale and impairment codes incorporated or referenced herein are the property of U B Foundation Activities, Inc. ©1993, 2001 U B Foundation Activities, Inc. The FIM mark is owned by UBFA, Inc.

39. FIM™ Instrument*

	ADMISSION	DISCHARGE	GOAL
SELF-CARE			
A. Eating	☐	☐	☐
B. Grooming	☐	☐	☐
C. Bathing	☐	☐	☐
D. Dressing - Upper	☐	☐	☐
E. Dressing - Lower	☐	☐	☐
F. Toileting	☐	☐	☐
SPHINCTER CONTROL			
G. Bladder	☐	☐	☐
H. Bowel	☐	☐	☐
TRANSFERS			
I. Bed, Chair, Whlchair	☐	☐	☐
J. Toilet	☐	☐	☐
K. Tub, Shower	☐	☐	☐

W - Walk
C - wheelChair
B - Both

	ADMISSION	DISCHARGE	GOAL
LOCOMOTION			
L. Walk/Wheelchair	☐☐	☐☐	☐
M. Stairs	☐	☐	☐

A - Auditory
V - Visual
B - Both

	ADMISSION	DISCHARGE	GOAL
COMMUNICATION			
N. Comprehension	☐☐	☐☐	☐
O. Expression	☐☐	☐☐	☐

V - Vocal
N - Nonvocal
B - Both

	ADMISSION	DISCHARGE	GOAL
SOCIAL COGNITION			
P. Social Interaction	☐	☐	☐
Q. Problem Solving	☐	☐	☐
R. Memory	☐	☐	☐

FIM LEVELS

No Helper
7 Complete Independence (Timely, Safely)
6 Modified Independence (Device)

Helper - Modified Dependence
5 Supervision (Subject = 100%)
4 Minimal Assistance (Subject = 75% or more)
3 Moderate Assistance (Subject = 50% or more)

Helper - Complete Dependence
2 Maximal Assistance (Subject = 25% or more)
1 Total Assistance (Subject less than 25%)

0 Activity does not occur; Use this code only at admission

OMB-0938-0842 (expires: 01-31-2003)

FORM F—cont'd

Continued

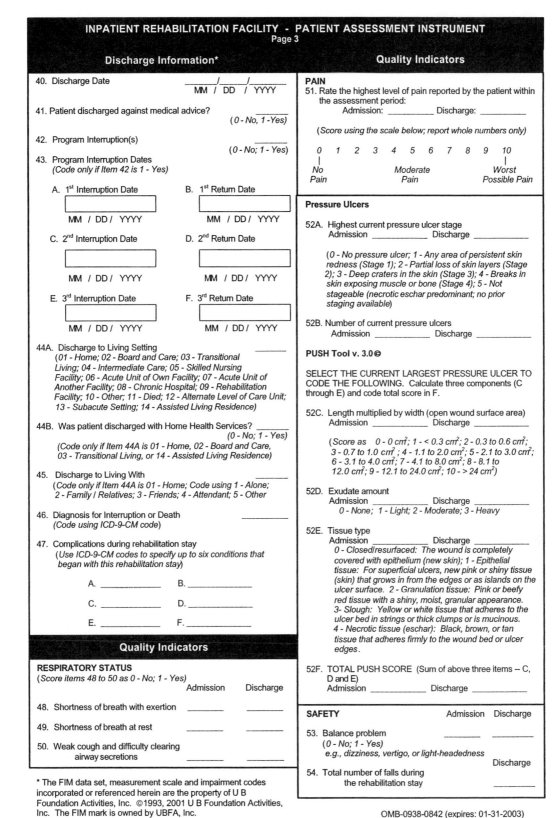

INPATIENT REHABILITATION FACILITY - PATIENT ASSESSMENT INSTRUMENT
Page 3

Discharge Information*

40. Discharge Date _____ / _____ / _____
MM / DD / YYYY

41. Patient discharged against medical advice? _____
(0 - No, 1 -Yes)

42. Program Interruption(s) _____
(0 - No; 1 - Yes)

43. Program Interruption Dates
(Code only if Item 42 is 1 - Yes)

A. 1st Interruption Date   B. 1st Return Date

MM / DD / YYYY   MM / DD / YYYY

C. 2nd Interruption Date   D. 2nd Return Date

MM / DD / YYYY   MM / DD / YYYY

E. 3rd Interruption Date   F. 3rd Return Date

MM / DD / YYYY   MM / DD / YYYY

44A. Discharge to Living Setting _____
(01 - Home; 02 - Board and Care; 03 - Transitional
Living; 04 - Intermediate Care; 05 - Skilled Nursing
Facility; 06 - Acute Unit of Own Facility; 07 - Acute Unit of
Another Facility; 08 - Chronic Hospital; 09 - Rehabilitation
Facility; 10 - Other; 11 - Died; 12 - Alternate Level of Care Unit;
13 - Subacute Setting; 14 - Assisted Living Residence)

44B. Was patient discharged with Home Health Services? _____
(0 - No; 1 - Yes)
(Code only if Item 44A is 01 - Home, 02 - Board and Care,
03 - Transitional Living, or 14 - Assisted Living Residence)

45. Discharge to Living With _____
(Code only if Item 44A is 01 - Home; Code using 1 - Alone;
2 - Family / Relatives; 3 - Friends; 4 - Attendant; 5 - Other)

46. Diagnosis for Interruption or Death _____
(Code using ICD-9-CM code)

47. Complications during rehabilitation stay
(Use ICD-9-CM codes to specify up to six conditions that
began with this rehabilitation stay)

A. _____   B. _____

C. _____   D. _____

E. _____   F. _____

Quality Indicators

RESPIRATORY STATUS
(Score items 48 to 50 as 0 - No; 1 - Yes)

	Admission	Discharge
48. Shortness of breath with exertion	_____	_____
49. Shortness of breath at rest	_____	_____
50. Weak cough and difficulty clearing airway secretions	_____	_____

Quality Indicators

PAIN

51. Rate the highest level of pain reported by the patient within the assessment period:
Admission: _____   Discharge: _____

(Score using the scale below; report whole numbers only)

0   1   2   3   4   5   6   7   8   9   10
| | |
No   Moderate   Worst
Pain   Pain   Possible Pain

Pressure Ulcers

52A. Highest current pressure ulcer stage
Admission _____   Discharge _____

(0 - No pressure ulcer; 1 - Any area of persistent skin
redness (Stage 1); 2 - Partial loss of skin layers (Stage
2); 3 - Deep craters in the skin (Stage 3); 4 - Breaks in
skin exposing muscle or bone (Stage 4); 5 - Not
stageable (necrotic eschar predominant; no prior
staging available)

52B. Number of current pressure ulcers
Admission _____   Discharge _____

PUSH Tool v. 3.0©

SELECT THE CURRENT LARGEST PRESSURE ULCER TO
CODE THE FOLLOWING. Calculate three components (C
through E) and code total score in F.

52C. Length multiplied by width (open wound surface area)
Admission _____   Discharge _____

(Score as   0 - 0 cm^2; 1 - < 0.3 cm^2; 2 - 0.3 to 0.6 cm^2;
3 - 0.7 to 1.0 cm^2 ; 4 - 1.1 to 2.0 cm^2; 5 - 2.1 to 3.0 cm^2;
6 - 3.1 to 4.0 cm^2; 7 - 4.1 to 8.0 cm^2; 8 - 8.1 to
12.0 cm^2; 9 - 12.1 to 24.0 cm^2; 10 - > 24 cm^2)

52D. Exudate amount
Admission _____   Discharge _____
0 - None; 1 - Light; 2 - Moderate; 3 - Heavy

52E. Tissue type
Admission _____   Discharge _____
0 - Closed/resurfaced: The wound is completely
covered with epithelium (new skin); 1 - Epithelial
tissue: For superficial ulcers, new pink or shiny tissue
(skin) that grows in from the edges or as islands on the
ulcer surface. 2 - Granulation tissue: Pink or beefy
red tissue with a shiny, moist, granular appearance.
3- Slough: Yellow or white tissue that adheres to the
ulcer bed in strings or thick clumps or is mucinous.
4 - Necrotic tissue (eschar): Black, brown, or tan
tissue that adheres firmly to the wound bed or ulcer
edges.

52F. TOTAL PUSH SCORE (Sum of above three items -- C,
D and E)
Admission _____   Discharge _____

SAFETY   Admission   Discharge

53. Balance problem   _____   _____
(0 - No; 1 - Yes)
e.g., dizziness, vertigo, or light-headedness
Discharge

54. Total number of falls during
the rehabilitation stay   _____

* The FIM data set, measurement scale and impairment codes
incorporated or referenced herein are the property of U B
Foundation Activities, Inc. ©1993, 2001 U B Foundation Activities,
Inc. The FIM mark is owned by UBFA, Inc.

OMB-0938-0842 (expires: 01-31-2003)

FORM F—cont'd

Index

Page references in *italics* indicate figures; those followed by *t* indicate tables.